# CHAIR VINYASA

*Yoga Flow for Every Body*

*The Instructor's Manual*

*By*

*Delia Quigley*

All instructions and sequences in this book are not intended to be a substitute for a trained health professional's guidance or counseling. Not all exercises are suitable for everyone and the exercises in this book may result in injury. Anyone using this book assumes the risk of injury resulting from performing these exercises. To reduce or prevent injury consult your doctor before beginning this or any other exercise program. The creator, and distributors of this book disclaim any liabilities or loss in connection with the exercise and advice herein.

# TABLE OF CONTENTS

# ACKNOWLEDGEMENTS

The source and inspiration for use of a folding chair is Sri B.K.S. Iyengar, the founder of Iyengar Yoga and a revered teacher throughout the world. It is with the deepest gratitude that I acknowledge the influence he has had on my yoga practice and life. From his teachings I have learned from many knowledgable yoga instructors who have guided their students with patience and understanding.

I am grateful to my teacher, Godfrey Devereux, founder of the Dynamic Yoga Training Method, who introduced me to the folding chair as a stabilizing prop. Coming from an aggressive Ashtanga yoga practice I was reluctant to accept a humble chair into my warrior practice. Once I did however, I was able to soften more deeply into poses, holding for longer and longer periods of time. As I have matured, I turn to the chair more often as a way to maintain the level of integrity I have achieved in my 32 years of practice.

My appreciation and thanks to Denise Kay, co-founder of Ha-Tha Yoga Method and good friend, for bringing her extensive knowledge, integrity, experience and humor to the creation of our Chair Yoga Certification program.

Denise is a highly respected yoga instructor in New Jersey bringing her special way of teaching to all of her classes. Without her, this book would not have been written and she continues to inspire me with her creative yoga work with each passing year.

My sincere thanks to Denise Kay, Kate McGuinness and John Fazio for posing for the photos in this book; and for Kate McGuinness and Shelly Mantegna's editing skills. I am grateful to have been a part of their personal transformation through the practice of yoga and now, as instructors, they assist others in a positive way. They are each wonderful role models.

And to all yoga practitioners and instructors exploring new possibilities for broken bodies and minds seeking to heal and grow stronger, I give thanks for the work that you do in the world.

Delia Quigley
Co-founder Ha-Tha Yoga Method

## WHY CHAIR VINYASA?

In the Ha-Tha Yoga Method, created by myself, Delia Quigley and Denise Kay, we teach the Five Techniques of Yoga: asana, pranayama, drishti, vinyasa and bandhas, to correspond to the Five Elements of Nature, earth, air, space, water and fire. We have experienced that this type of practice allows for a deeper mind-body integration and provides a safe, more effective practice.

Vinyasa does not have to be a fast paced, sweat inducing experience. In fact moving too fast with no awareness can cause injuries to the body due to instability and misalignment. In the 8-Limbs of Yoga, asana is the third limb on the path; and according to Patanjali, the author of The Yoga Sutras, not entirely a very important step. It is practiced to prepare the body for more intense breath work (pranayama), which takes the practitioner deeper into concentration, (dharana), graduating to meditation (dhyana), and finally to liberation (samadhi).

In the few sutras about asana that Patanjali mentions he tells us that *sthira* and *sukham asanam* are necessary; in other words the practitioner needs to be stable and comfortable in each pose. This requires a slower paced practice with longer holding of the postures. However, this does not negate the positive attributes of a Vinyasa flow between each sequence of asanas.

In Chair Vinyasa there is time to stay and hold each pose (Earth element), to engage the Bandhas (Fire element), to connect the body-mind through breath awareness (Air element), to do so with full awareness (Space element), and to soften through movement as a Vinyasa flow (Water element).

In this way, any level of practitioner, even novice students, can benefit from this simple yet safe and effective yoga prop. This book is written for yoga instructors and other body and mental health trainers interested in introducing clients to yoga with knowledge and integrity.

It is recommended that you have practiced yoga and/or been certified as a yoga teacher to fully understand the purpose and explanations for each pose.

Yoga students can use this book to further enhance your practice, but it is also recommended that you practice under the guidance of a certified instructor when and where possible. Most of all this book is written to bring attention to a simple prop, a folding chair, that can be used to enhance and further deepen your experience as a yoga practitioner.

# INTRODUCTION

Yoga is booming! In 2015 statistics show that there are 15 million people practicing yoga; 72.2 % are female, 40% are 35-54 years old with 18.4% of students over 55 years of age. That brings a wide range of students coming to yoga classes looking for a way to stretch, strengthen, relax, and, for some, to sweat.

No one attends a yoga class expecting to be injured, but it is all too common these days. Often the body is expected to speed through poses in extreme heat pushing to keep up rather than the practitioner learning to be sensitive to what the body is actually willing or able to do in the moment.

I have been teaching yoga for 32 years and have worked with all ages and types of bodies. Many people today are broken, either physically, mentally, emotionally or spiritually. You come to yoga looking for relief from the stress of life and that is exactly what you should find. This can happen with a vinyasa flow style or restorative class, and for many students the use of a single prop, such as a folding chair, can make the difference between stable and supportive or stressful and dangerous.

The practice of Hatha Yoga is designed to engage the body-mind in an inquiry based on sensation, the language your body uses to communicate.

To listen and understand what your body is asking in a pose requires time, awareness and an internal focus. In this way the ego-mind is subdued, calming the aggressive desire to push, pull, and demand from the physical body what can in time weaken, tear and injure.

A chair provides a stable support allowing you to hold poses longer resulting in a deeper flexibility and strength. In the holding, your body-mind can soften, shift and move deeper into the pose. For many to progress in yoga practice, this sensitivity and time are essential to a safe and effective practice.

On the other hand, when you are moving too quickly through a sequence of poses, precision of alignment is difficult to find. Your body has little time to adapt bone, muscle, tendon and sinew in the rush from one pose to the next.

This is where the toes begin to grip the floor seeking a "toe hold" because there is not enough time to ground the feet properly. The mind becomes tense, the jaw locks in a grimace and the core of the body hardens. Bad habits form and when injury occurs, yoga gets the blame.

The folding chair as a yoga prop is a part of the Iyengar way of teaching yoga; however it is gaining in popularity in yoga studios, particularly by supporting the limited movement of senior citizens and those with physical injury.

You might find these listed under a "Gentle Yoga Class", or "Seniors Chair Yoga". However, this important prop can also be beneficial for intermediate and advanced students looking to take their practice to the next level.

I have been exploring a Vinyasa Flow using the folding chair to move slowly from one asana to another. Consider the use of a ballet barre in classical training. The first hour of a ballet class is spent working at the barre to ensure stability and to better develop flexibility and muscle strength while maintaining proper alignment. So why not use the folding chair in the same way?

I feel that a chair will fast become the number one yoga prop in yoga studios and therefore, training is essential for instructors. Chair Yoga training can benefit certified yoga instructors, teachers-in-training, mental health counselors, physical therapists and experienced yoga students.

In this book you will learn to bring the benefits of yoga to your students utilizing yoga poses, breath and total relaxation with the support of a folding chair.

In the Ha-Tha Yoga Method Training, we place an emphasis on providing instructors with the tools of knowledge and experience to better create a yoga class based upon their student's physical, emotional and mental needs, whether novice, beginner, intermediate or advanced practitioners.

If you would like more information please view our website:
ha-thayogamethod.com
hathayogamethod@gmail.com

_____

## CHAIR CONSIDERATIONS

There are a number of things to take into consideration when using a chair for use as a prop.

### PURCHASE

**Have** two folding chairs, one with a padded seat and upper back rest and another with the back rest removed and no seat padding.

**Height** of the chair should be considered for proper alignment and not cause too much strain or tension in the muscles. a) Sitting on the chair, make sure your knees align with the hips and feet are fully grounded to the floor. b) Check that the back of the chair supports a straight spine.

**Padding** on the chair seat and back rest provide a cushion for older and broken bodies.

### PROPS

**Props** such as blocks, straps, blankets, wedges, and bolsters can be used to
a) lengthen the arms  b) prop up the hips
c) create more stability d) hold a pose longer e) support the opening of chest and back.

**Blocks** can be used to provide height to a students legs or extra extension for the arms.

**Folded** blankets or yoga mats can be used to lift the pelvis and pad the chair seat and upper back.

### PLACEMENT

**3-8** chairs can be arranged front, sides and back to support individuals with stability issues. This prevents wasting energy moving the chair from one position to another.

**To** prevent blankets from slipping cut a 12"x12" piece of no slip rug pad or old yoga mat and place it on the seat or back rest under the blanket.

**For** vinyasa flow placement of the chair can be to the front, back or side of mat.

**Depending** on the pose the seat can be turned towards or away from the student.

**Remember** that a chair is a movable object and awareness is called for when shifting the body from pose to pose.

**Holding** poses allows the muscles, when stretched, to gradually release as a relaxation response begins to dominate. This can take from 30 seconds to 2 minutes to occur. Let your body be your guide.

**Use** the chair under the guidance of a certified yoga instructor who has knowledge of the use of the chair.

## TYPES OF CHAIRS

The conventional metal folding chair as seen to the right, is most commonly used in Iyengar style yoga. The chairs have been adapted for yoga poses by removing the back rest and the bottom front rung. The chair to the far right has lengthened legs for taller students and the front rung has been left in place, though set higher on the legs.

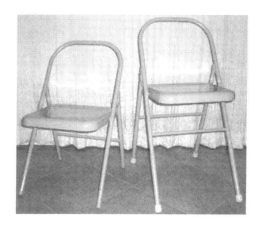

The single backed chair to the right has a padded seat and back and is constructed of a high grade steel for strength and weight bearing. It is more comfortable for Seniors as the padding acts as a cushion for the body. This style is available in most department stores and the back rest can be removed by a qualified welder to create a wide enough opening for reclining poses.

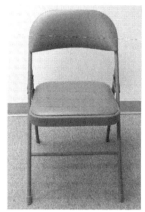

The third chair on the right has been specifically designed for yoga poses and includes a detachable addition to better support back bending poses. The seat is padded as is the back rest. The front rung is placed higher on the legs. This allows the head to rest comfortably under the front edge of the chair.

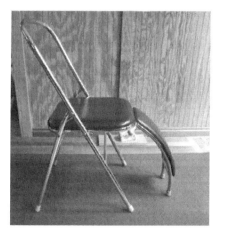

Arrange the chairs as you see to the right, to support a flow of poses or to create more stability for individuals needing to hold on to a sturdy object. This benefits those with Multiple Sclerosis, Parkinson's disease, arthritis and those recovering from hip and knee replacements.

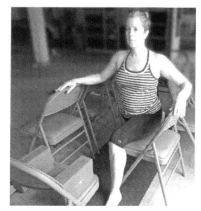

## HISTORY

Sri Krishnamacharya, who is one of our biggest influences in yoga today, taught students individually. One of Krishnamacharya's students was his brother in-law, B.K.S. Iyengar. Iyengar began studying with Krishnamacharya as a young boy. As a boy, he was quite sickly and as he began practicing yoga his health improved. He used yoga to heal himself and was completely convinced that if he put his mind to it he would be able to devise methods of healing others.

B.K.S. Iyengar introduced the folding chair to his students as a means to bring stability to the body-mind, while allowing the body to properly align in each asana. He also used various props to provide practitioners access to the benefits of postures regardless of physical condition, age, or length of study. In this way it became therapeutic.

Props help all students, even the advanced practitioner, to accomplish poses with precision and to gain the benefit of the posture. They allow students to hold a pose longer, allowing time to investigate the quality of the posture in greater depth. The folding chair was introduced for this purpose.

According to his son, T.K.V. Desikachar, "What makes my father unique was his insistence on attending to each individual and to his or her uniqueness. If we respect each individually, it naturally means we will always start from where each person currently is. The starting point is never the teacher's needs but those of the student." Through working with the chair, we can meet everyones needs as individuals.

———————

## STUDENTS WHO BENEFIT

### Use of the chair benefits:

- Students who are elderly
- Students with knee and or hip issues
- Students with issues of balance
- Students who are overweight
- Students with MS
- Students with Parkinson's
- Students with other neuromuscular diseases
- Novice & Beginner students
- Intermediate students wanting to find alignment and advance

## SENIORS

**The world's senior population is growing rapidly** as is their interest in leading healthy and active lives. On the whole, we are living longer and looking for programs that will support us during our older years. Aging can slow us down as we tend to do less, becoming more susceptible to ailments, weight gain, arthritis and disease. The less we move, the more susceptible we become to a variety of ailments, and so it becomes a truly vicious cycle.

**Yoga has been shown to** help alleviate or reduce many of these health challenges, making it an increasingly popular exercise choice for our older adult population.

**Chair yoga provides** therapeutic benefits for older individuals who may not be able to stand for long periods of time or who may be uncomfortable moving up and down off the floor. Many standard yoga poses can easily be adapted for seniors to perform while sitting in a chair.

### Benefits when using a chair

- May increase circulation in the feet, legs, knees, hips, shoulders and elbows, which helps the general well-being of the physical body
- Helps arthritis, back pain, blood pressure, osteoporosis and many other physical issues
- Helps heart and lung functions. (The breathing techniques used in yoga are very effective for people with emphysema and asthma and aid in heart function)
- May improve mental clarity - Following the directions and guidance of a yoga teacher challenges the brain and supports the mind/body connection for better mental processing
- Helps support better sleep with learning how to regulate the breath, and through relaxation techniques

---

## KNEE ISSUES

### If guided correctly knee injuries can benefit from gentle yoga:

- Everyday joint pain
- Torn meniscus
- Torn ACL (anterior cruciate ligament) PCL (posterior cruciate ligament)
- Arthritis

### Every day joint pain can be caused by:

- Overuse
- Underuse
- Too much sugar

### What a yoga instructor should know:

- The student's exact health issue
- Does their doctor know the student is beginning a yoga practice?
- Has the student had knee surgery and if so, how long ago was their surgery?
- Are they being treated and what type of treatment are they getting?
- What are their restrictions?
- What are their limitations?
- What is the student's goal? (To gain extension, flexion or both)

## KNEE REPLACEMENT

**When less invasive treatments fail** some will opt for a knee joint replacement. Those who undergo a knee replacement may want to incorporate yoga into part of their post-surgery healing regimen.

But unless it's done carefully and with appropriate modifications, yoga could make knees feel worse.

After surgery, the replacement knee is expected to allow between 120 and 155 degrees of flexion. The knee will not bend as much as a healthier and more flexible one, so care is needed when working with the knee replacement.

### What a yoga instructor should know:

- How long ago was the surgery? After any surgery it is recommended waiting 6 to 8 weeks
- Make sure they have their doctor's approval
- People with knee replacements need to be especially careful about alignment
- Protect knees by keeping them aligned with the ankles and hips
- Yoga will help students strengthen hips, thighs, calves, and ankles
- When beginning with someone new, keep it simple and avoid strain on the knee
- Avoid any twist in the knee or ankle such as in Garudasana, Eagle pose. Use chair modifications for poses
- Be cautious when doing a deep knee bend that is held for a long amount of time
- Check in with the student, throughout the class, to see how they are feeling
- Standing poses will strengthen the hamstrings and quadriceps, which often become weak after surgery

# TOTAL HIP REPLACEMENT (THR)

**A total hip replacement** (THR) is a surgical procedure whereby the diseased connective tissue (cartilage) and bone of the hip joint are surgically replaced with artificial materials. The hip joint is a ball and socket joint. The ball is the head of the thigh bone (femur). The socket (acetabulum) is a cup-shaped indentation in the pelvis.

During hip replacement surgery, the head of the femur is removed and replaced with a metal ball set on a stem. The stem is inserted into the canal of the femur. It may be fixed in place with cement, or the stem may be designed for placement without bone cement. The socket is sanded down to healthy bone, and a plastic cup or socket is held in place with screws, bone cement or the ball to socket pressure.

**Traditional surgery**, the surgeons access the joint area through the upper thigh, either through the lateral (outside) part or the posterior (back) part. During the surgery, the surgeon must detach several major muscles from the pelvis or femur (thigh bone), in order to reach the hip joint. The detached muscles must then be reattached after the new joint is in place. Because the entry point is in the rear (literally!), this is called posterior hip replacement.

**The latest surgical approach is an** anterior hip replacement, which is gaining popularity because it spares the muscles and allows quicker recovery time.

This procedure is performed with the patient lying on his or her back on a specially designed surgical table. This position lets the surgeon access the joint from the front of the hip area without surgically detaching any muscles. Instead, the hip joint is reached through naturally occurring openings between the muscles.

**Working with a student who has had a hip replacement**

Proper exercise after surgery, such as yoga, can reduce stiffness, increase flexibility and muscle strength. How much and how soon are dependent on the student's physical health before surgery and the presence of chronic conditions that may affect the speed of recovery.

As technology has advanced, so too the number of years prosthetic parts can be relied upon to serve their purpose. It is now more common to see hip replacements in younger people, who may be in better overall physical condition and who will heal faster.

_____

## If the surgery was Anterior approach:

The conservative cautions are opposite to those for the posterior approach:

- Limited abduction (separating legs at wide angle) for 6 months
- Limited external rotation (turning thighs out) for 6 months
- Limited extension (stretching backward) of the hip joint for one year

## If the surgery was Posterior approach:

- No adduction (crossing the affected leg past the midline of the body) for 3 months, and limited adduction for another 3 months after that.
- No internal rotation for 3 months, and limited internal rotation for another 3 months after that.
- No flexion past 90 degrees for 6 months, and limited flexion past 90 degrees for another 6 months after that.
- No postures such as Child's pose, Eagle pose, Pigeon pose and many others.

Warrior postures need to be adjusted to student's ability. In Warrior II, emphasis on internal rotation of back leg needs to be altered. External rotation of the front leg needs to be modified as well.

Any of these movements could put the hip at risk for dislocation, or at the very least disturb the healing process, especially during the first few months after surgery.

Even though no muscles are detached or compromised while replacing a hip joint, there are definitely some incisions being made that affect other support structures: e.g., ligaments and the joint capsule.

So major modifications are in order for poses like *Parsva Virabhadrasana*, Side Warrior (which involves abduction and external rotation) and *Raja Kapotasana*, King Pigeon (back leg's hip joint is in extension) for the affected hip.

## What you need to ask:

How long ago was the surgery?

Does your doctor know you are taking yoga classes?

Was the surgery Posterior or Anterior?

———————————

# MULTIPLE SCLEROSIS (MS)

**MS involves** an immune mediated process in which an abnormal response to the body's immune system is directed against the central nervous system, which is made up of the brain, spinal cord and optical nerves.

Within the central nervous system, the immune system attacks myelin - the fatty substance that surrounds and insulates the nerve fibers, as well as the nerve fibers themselves. This damages the myelin sheath forming scar tissue (sclerosis), giving it's name.

When any part of the myelin sheath or nerve fiber is damaged or destroyed, nerve impulses traveling to and from the brain and the spinal cord are distorted or interrupted, producing a wide variety of symptoms.

## Exercise

**Exercise offers** many benefits for people with MS. In addition to improving overall health, certain types of exercise reduce fatigue and improve bladder and bowl function, body strength, and mood. More and more MS experts note that yoga, with its emphasis on relaxation, breathing, stretching and deliberate movement, is a good choice of exercise.

Stretching exercises reduce stiffness and increase mobility. Chair yoga can be a part of an exercise plan for someone with MS' abilities and limitations.

**How yoga can help:**

- Poses and breathing techniques focus the mind on the body
- Non-competitive and adaptable
- Benefits posture and balance
- Educates about muscles and how to strengthen and stretch
- Helps release tension in the body allowing for more energy
- Uses relaxation techniques to reduce stress

---

## PARKINSON'S DISEASE (PD)

**Parkinson's Disease** causes certain brain cells to die. These are the cells that help control movement and coordination. The disease leads to shaking (tremors) and trouble walking and moving.

Nerve cells use the brain chemical dopamine to help control muscle movement. With Parkinson's, the brain cells that control movement cannot send messages to the muscles, making it hard to control them. Science has yet to discover what causes these brain cells to waste away.

*Exercise is beneficial for individuals with Parkinson's and should be considered a standard part of treatment. Beyond the benefits to physical health and mood, new research in animals shows that physical exercise may even protect the health of existing dopamine cells -- and the same may be true for humans.*

**Yoga may be the perfect exercise** for Parkinson's patients because of its gentle and slow movements. The *Parkinson's Hope Digest* reports that a number of Parkinson' patients have reported diminished symptoms and improved motion and emotional spirits after taking yoga classes.

## How yoga can help:

• Stretching the body may help improve mobility and range of motion

• Yoga classes incorporate balance training and back strengthening postures, shoulder movements and meditation

• Yoga also stresses the importance of proper breathing techniques to enhance lung function

• The practice of yoga can improve muscle strength and increase mobility

• The various yoga poses can lessen Parkinson's symptoms and enhance both physical and mental strength

• Yoga can have an uplifting emotional impact on people with Parkinson's

———————————

# STROKE

**A stroke (or "brain attack")** occurs when part of the brain stops receiving the steady supply of oxygen-rich blood it needs. This can happen because of a blockage in a vessel supplying blood to the brain, or because a blood vessel in the brain breaks. Either way, the shut-off damages fragile brain tissue.

The effect of the damage depends on what part of the brain is affected. A stroke can interfere with speech, cause memory problems, or effect the movement of the arms or legs on one side of the body. Stroke can also lead to difficulty with balance and increase the risk of falls.

There are 2 types of strokes:

**Ischemic Stroke**: is caused by a blockage of blood flow to a certain part of the brain.

**Hemorrhagic**: this occurs when a blood vessel inside the brain ruptures allowing blood to pool inside or around healthy brain tissue. In many cases this is caused by high blood pressure.

**How yoga can help:**

**In recent studies** yoga has been found to be a useful tool for people recovering from strokes.

In an 8 week adapted yoga program, stroke survivors were found to have a greater improvement in balance, flexibility, strength and endurance because it helped with neuromuscular control.

**What you need to know:**

Since stroke patients display a variety of physical limitations you will need to:

- Be certain that the student has consulted with their doctor
- Understand the individual's limitations and work with and around those limitations
- Make sure the student is secure in his/her balance
- Use balance and strengthening postures
- Use pranayama for relaxation

———————————

## OBESITY

**Obesity is a medical condition** in which excess body fat has accumulated to the extent that it may have an adverse effect on health. It is the excess of fat on the body which causes several diseases:

- High blood pressure
- Diabetes
- Heart disease
- Sleep apnea
- Certain types of cancer
- Osteoarthritis
- Infertility

**Obesity is usually caused by:**

- Overeating
- Lack of physical activity
- A low energy level, which leads to inactivity

Yoga can help, but one should begin slowly by using props such as the chair, blocks and blankets.

**How yoga can help:**
- By improving the body's alignment to reduce strain on ligaments and joints

- Lowers blood pressure

- Supports weight loss

- Provides a connection between mind and body, which increases the self-esteem of an individual

- Helps one to understand the self better, becoming more conscious of food and diet

- Helps to fight depression, lifting mood

- Helps manage type 2 diabetes, by stabilizing blood sugar levels

New students should begin slowly as body size may impede poses that require bending or supporting weight.

**Using a chair in yoga can:**
- Take stress off taxed joints

- Help build self-esteem

- Provide insight to proper body alignment, breathing and mind patterns

- Strengthen and inspire a student to partake in other types of yoga or other activities which will continue to support weight loss

---

# NOTES

# ASANA

# STANDING POSES

Tadasana
Uttanasana
Anjanyasana
Marjaryasana Svanasana
Adho Mukha Svanasana
Trikonasana
Parivritta Trikonasana
Virabhadrasana I
Parsva Virabhadrasana
Triang Virabhadrasana
Parsvakonasana
Parsvottanasana
Prasarita Padottanasana

The asanas (poses) in Chair Vinyasa are arranged in a sequential order to better assist the practitioner in creating a comfortable vinyasa flow practice. We begin with standing poses to strengthen legs, open hips, lengthen hamstrings and extend the spine.

A vinyasa flow can begin from Tadasana, the mountain pose, or it can begin from a simple seated pose taking a moment to internalize the awareness and prepare for the flow of movement to breath.

Standing poses are strengthening, grounding, empowering asanas that help to focus the mind, connect to the breath and bring the student into the present moment.

# TADASANA
## Mountain Pose

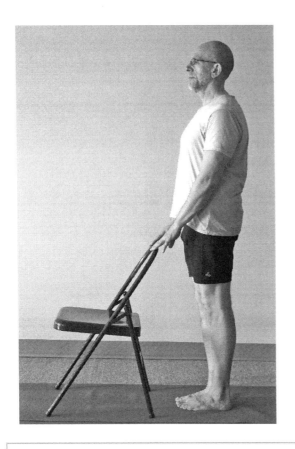 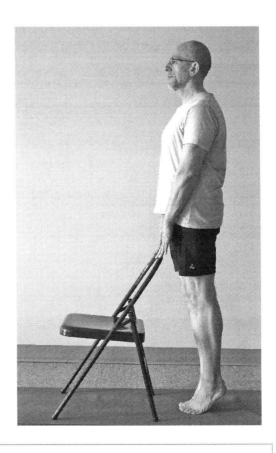

1. Stand with feet slightly apart.
2. Ground all four corners of the feet to the floor: base of the big toe, little toe, inner heel, outer heel.
3. Legs and back straight, shoulders down, hands lightly touching the back of the chair.
4. Gaze forward.
5. Take a moment to breathe and feel the balance of weight between the feet.

6. Gently press into the balls of the feet and lift the heels off the floor. Think of going up instead of forward with the body.
7. Lower the heels slowly and repeat, lifting and lowering for 5 repetitions.
8. Maintain contact with the chair, then try lifting the heels without touching the chair.

**NOTES**

*The feet are the foundation for standing asanas and attention should be paid to their alignment to ensure stability in a pose.*

*Remember that whatever is in contact to the floor or seat of the chair forms the foundation on which to build each yoga pose.*

# TADASANA VARIATIONS

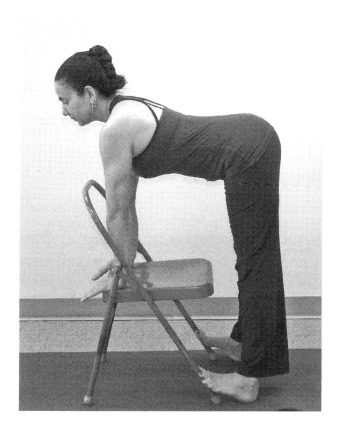 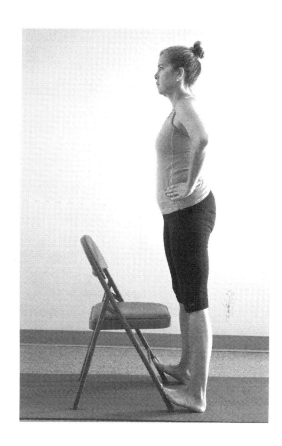

1. Lean forward and place hands on chair seat.
2. Place the ball of the foot along the front leg of the chair and stay in this position or come to standing with hands on hips.

3. Hold the pose for 5 breaths then slowly come forward place hands on chair to support the balance while removing feet from the chair leg.

**Notes**
*Wonderful stretch for the feet, calf muscles and the achilles tendon.*

# UTTANASANA
## Forward Bending Pose

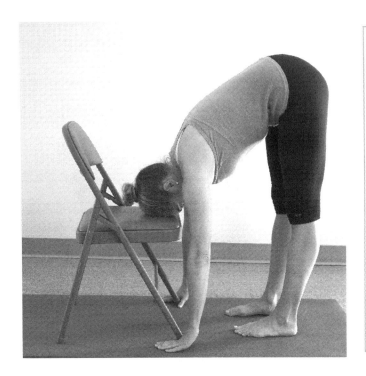

1. Inhale arms arise, exhale fold forward placing hands and forehead on chair seat.
2. Knees can be bent and straighten once into the pose.
3. Hands can rest on the chair or arms can be extended to the floor.
4. Hold the pose for 5 breaths.
5. Roll up through the spine to a standing position.

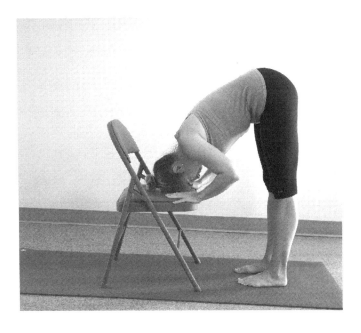

**NOTES**

*This pose can be done standing in front of the chair or sitting on the chair.*

*Arms can extend to the floor and/or hands can take hold of the chair leg when coming forward when sitting.*

*Bending the knees allows for the back to extend comfortably. Keep knees bent if hamstrings are tight and limiting back extension.*

# UTTANASANA VARIATIONS

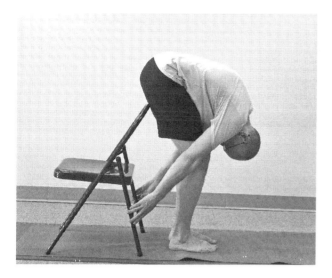

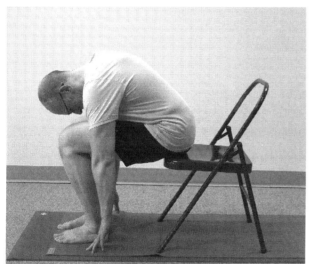

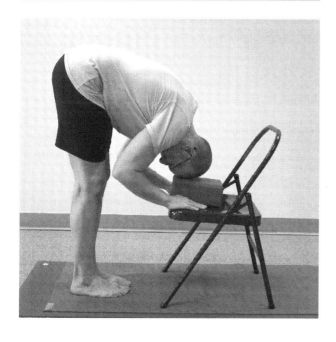

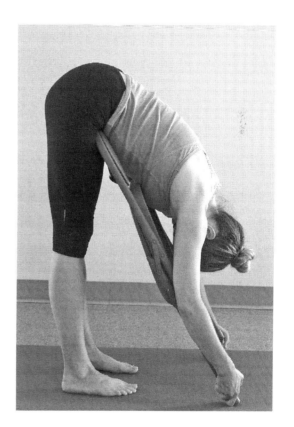

# ANJANYASANA
## Crescent Moon Pose

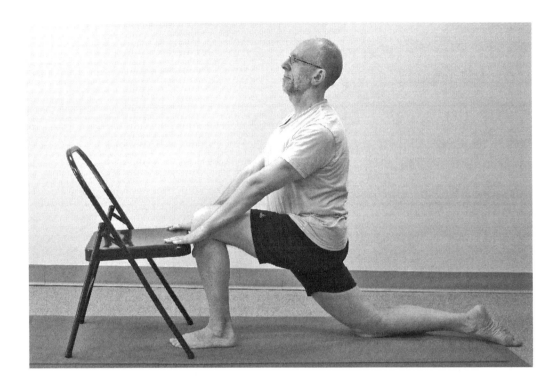

1. Step one leg back into a lunge holding to the front of the chair seat.
2. Lift the spine, lower the shoulders and gaze forward.
3. Ground the four corners of the front foot and lengthen the spine.
4. Maintain the alignment of right and left hips.
5. Keep the back leg extended in a straight line. Hold for 5 breaths.
6. To come out of the pose tuck the back toes, extend the leg and step the foot forward. Repeat on other side.

**NOTES**

The Anjanyasana variations demonstrate the hands placed higher on the back of the chair and with the chair placed to the side of the mat.

Revolving Anjanyasana provides stability as the body moves into a deep twist. Continue to maintain proper foot and knee alignment to support this stability.

# ANJANYASANA VARIATIONS

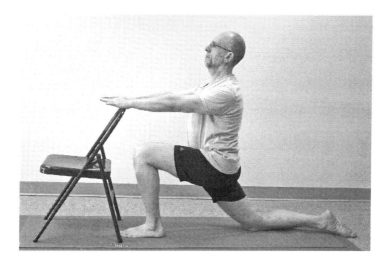

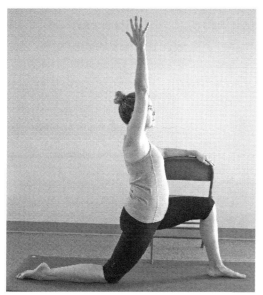

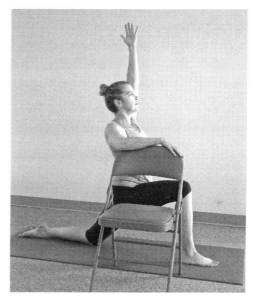

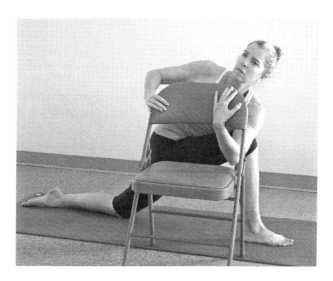

# MARJARYASAN SVANASANA
## Cat Dog Pose

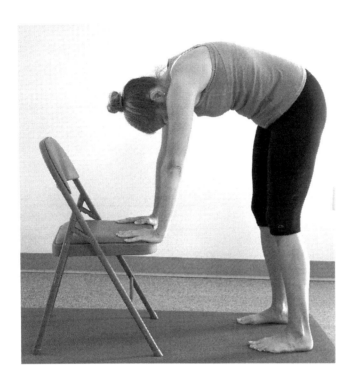

1. Place hands shoulder width apart on the seat of chair. Align the shoulders over the wrists and hips over the ankles.
2. Inhale and tilt the pelvis upwards. Gently round the back tucking the chin to the chest by the end of the movement.
3. Follow by tilting the pelvis downwards gently arching the back and looking slightly up and forward with the head.
4. Initiating the movement from the pelvis repeat 4-5 times.
5. Come to a neutral position before rolling up to a standing position.

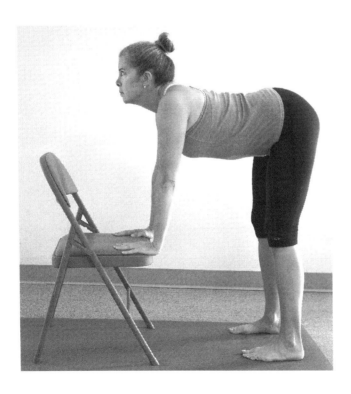

**NOTES**

*Be careful not to exaggerate rounding the upper back or force the arch in the lower back. Instead allow the movement of the pelvis to dictate the rounding and arching of the vertebrae.*

*Arms should remain straight with elbows soft, knees slightly bent to allow for more freedom of movement in the pelvic area.*

*The head is the last to arrive into position. Think of it as a wave that begins in the tailbone and moves up the spine to the crown of the head.*

# MARJARYASAN SVANASANA VARIATIONS

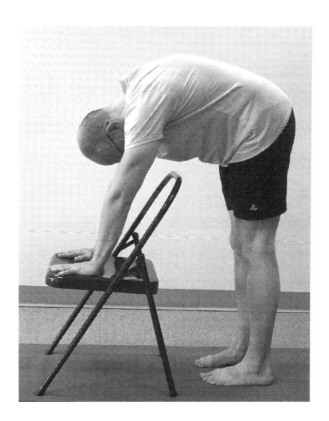

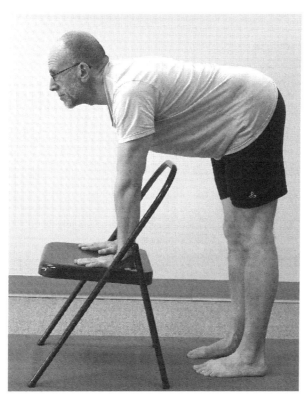

# ADHO MUKHA SVANASANA
## Downward Facing Dog Pose

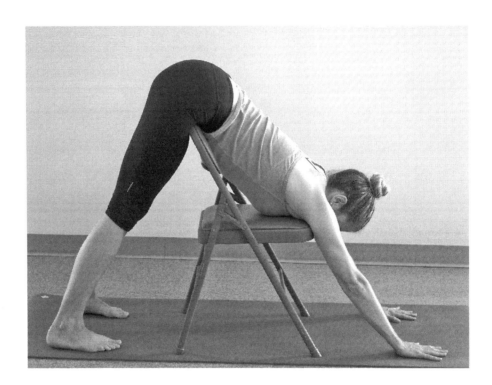

1. Place hands on chair seat and rest the hips along the top edge of the chair back.
2. Extend hands down and out to the floor bringing the front edge of the chair seat to the under arms and the chin forward of the seat.
3. Heels can be lifted to release tight hamstrings.
4. Keep the hips lifting away from the shoulders and gently extend the heels towards the floor.
5. Hold for 5 breaths.

**Notes**

*Extension of the back should be the focus of this asana. This variation allows for the lift in the hips and length in the back while taking weight off the hands.*

**Props**

*A blanket or folded mat placed under the hips can make the pose more comfortable.*

*Blocks placed under the hands or feet can provide lift if the chair is too tall or in need of more extension.*

# ADHO MUKHA SVANASANA VARIATIONS

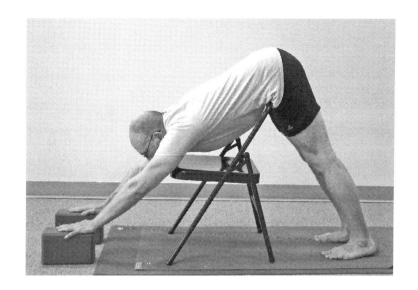

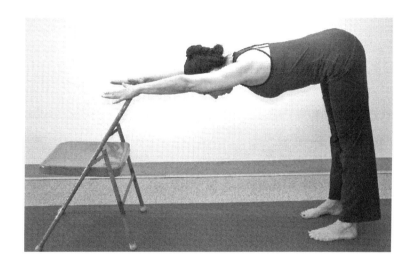

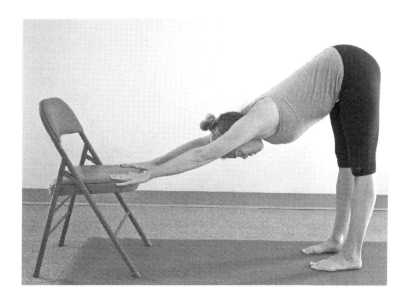

# TRIKONASANA
## Triangle Pose

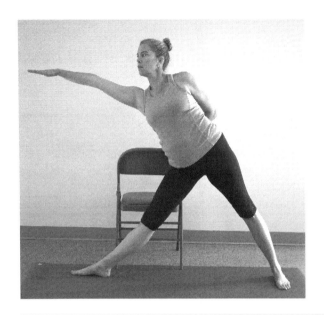 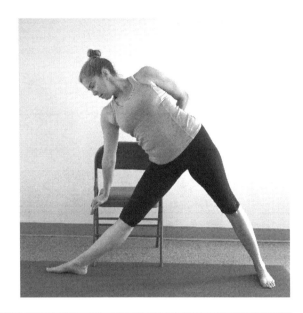

1. Step the feet out wide and align hips with the long edge of the mat.
2. Turn the right foot out 90 degrees and the left foot in 15 degrees.
3. Draw the right hip back slightly and extend the right arm out over the right foot.
4. Bring the right hand to the far corner of the chair seat. Continue to rotate the trunk of the body open and take the left hand to the upper back of the chair.
5. Slowly move the right hand lower on the chair rung maintaining the rotation and stability.

**NOTE:** *Holding the chair back allows for opening in the chest and shoulder as the body lowers towards the leg.*

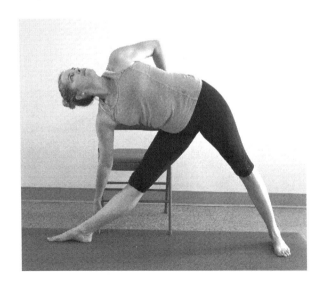 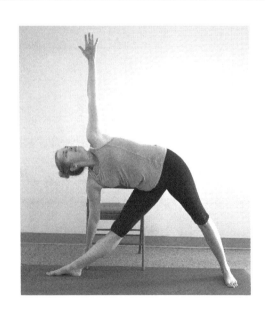

# TRIKONASANA VARIATIONS

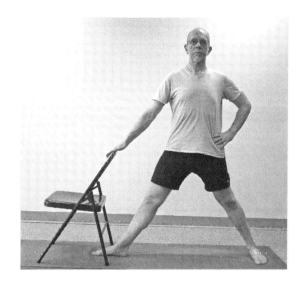 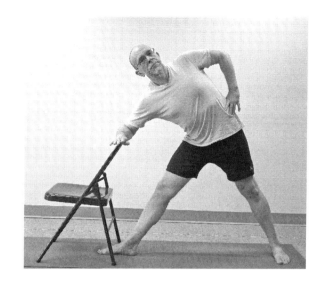

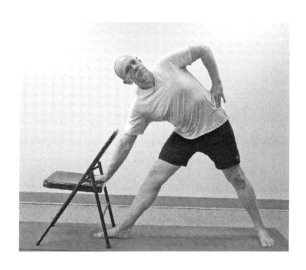 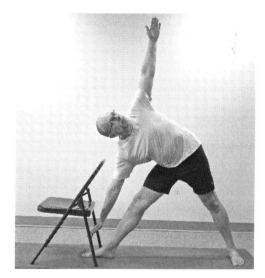

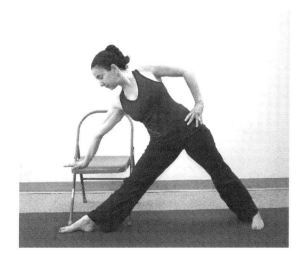 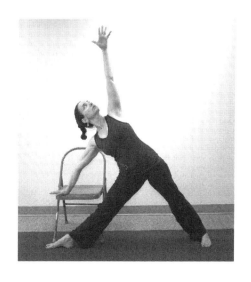

# PARIVRTTA TRIKONASANA
## Revolving Triangle Pose

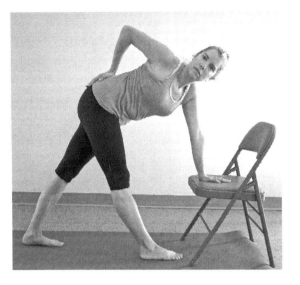
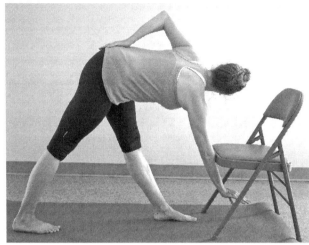

1. Align the legs on two planes with right foot front and knees straight.
2. Place the left hand on the center of chair seat and right hand on lower back. Revolve the upper body towards the right.
3. Hold or lower the hand to the chair rung and continue to revolve to the right side. Hold for 5 breaths and repeat on other side.

**NOTES**

*Reverse chair and place the hand on the upper edge of the chair back, then lower hand to the seat.*

*To align the hips bring the right hip back and up as the left hip comes forward and down.*

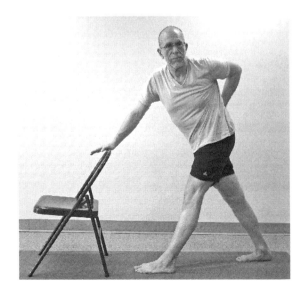
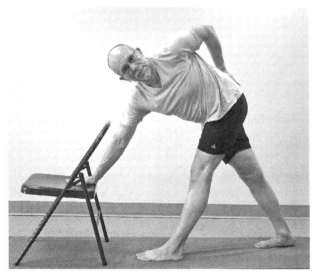

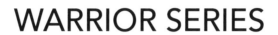

# WARRIOR SERIES

# VIRABHADRASANA I
## Warrior Pose

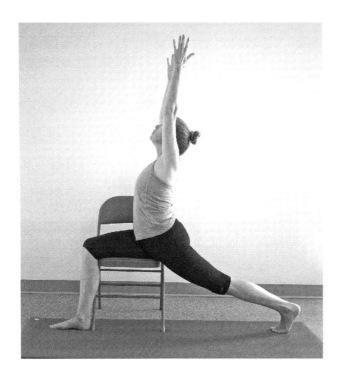

1. Sit the right thigh onto chair seat close to the front edge with back of knee against the edge of chair seat.
2. Extend the left leg grounding through the ball of the foot and straightening the knee.
3. Align the right knee over the right ankle keeping the foot facing forward and hips aligned.
4. Sit down onto the chair or lift up slightly to engage the right thigh.
5. Extend the arms up towards the ceiling and gaze to the thumbs.
6. Rotate the back foot inwards 35 degrees and lower the heel to the floor. Focus on extending into the outer heel to assist the left hip moving forward.
7. Hold for 5 breaths then repeat on the other side.

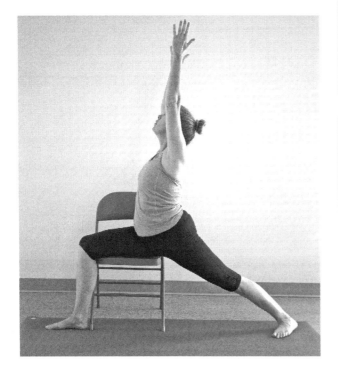

**PROPS**

*Allow the back leg to bend, place a block under the knee for support.*

*If chair seat is too low place a folded blanket or cushion under the thigh and adjust for individual stretch.*

*If the chair seat is too high place a block under the front foot to provide lift and proper alignment.*

# VIRABHADRASANA VARIATIONS

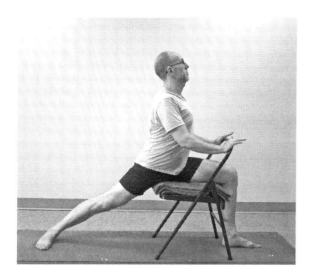 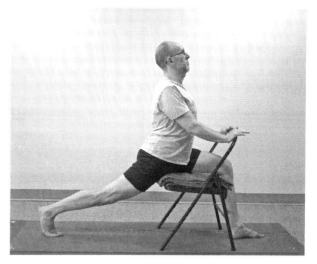

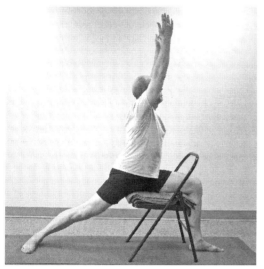 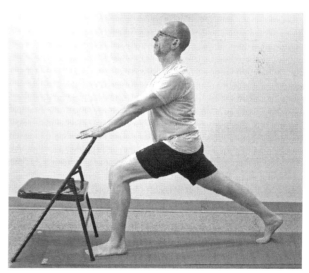

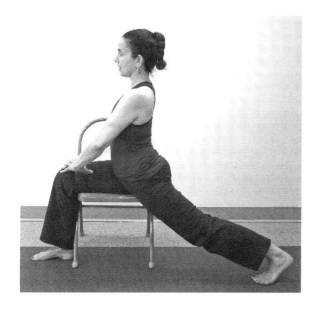 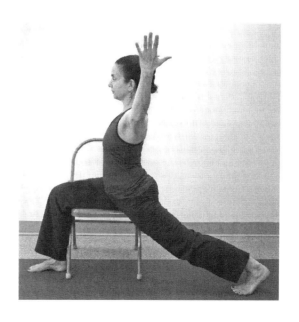

# PARSVA VIRABHADRASANA
## Side Warrior Pose

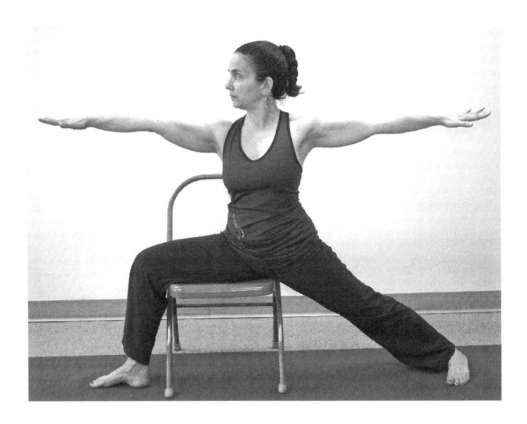

1. Sit the right thigh onto chair seat, knee to the edge.
2. Extend the left leg out to the side.
3. Hips align to the long edge of the mat.
4. Arms extend out to the sides aligning with the shoulders.
5. Ground the base of the right big toe, little toe, outer heel to align the knee.
6. Ground the base of the left big toe, inner heel to outer heel to align the hips.
7. Gaze is to the finger tips.
8. Hold for 5 breaths, then repeat on the other side.

**PROPS**

If the chair seat is too low place a folded blanket or cushion under the thigh and adjust for individual stretch.

If the chair seat is too high place a block under the front and back feet to provide lift and proper alignment.

# PARSVA VIRABHADRASANA VARIATIONS

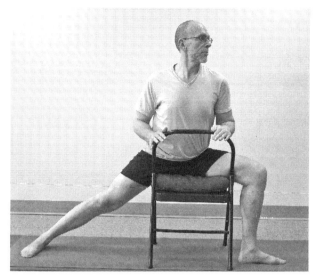
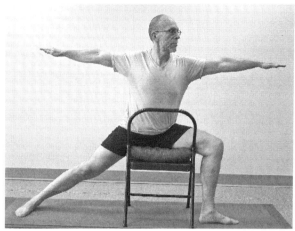

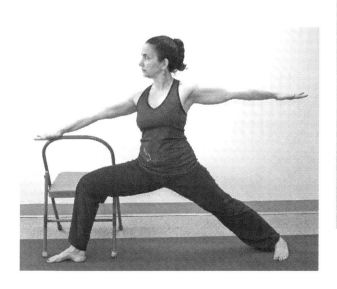

## NOTES

This is a difficult pose for students with tight hips, as it requires a deep sitting and extension in the groin and hips.

Feel free to prop with a blanket or cushion to provide more height or a block under the feet to give more lift.

The student can also lift up off the chair to engage the legs.

The extended leg can be be moved forward to accommodate the hips or slightly bent.

The last two photos demonstrate use of the chair that seems easier for most bodies to align properly.

# TRIANG VIRABHADRASANA
## Three Limb Warrior Pose

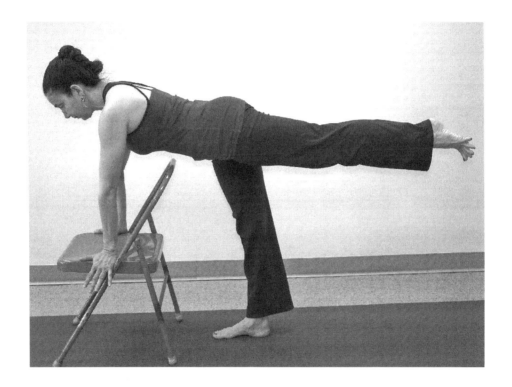

1. Place hands on outer edges of chair seat.
2. Align feet under hips and shift weight onto right foot extending left leg out behind.
3. Align hips parallel to the floor.
4. Begin to raise the back leg and gradually lift higher as flexibility allows.
5. Maintain weight on the standing leg, staying light on the hands.
6. Bring the body into a parallel alignment to the floor and gaze forward.
7. Think of extension rather than height of the leg.

---

**NOTES**

*The challenge is to keep the hip of the extended leg in alignment with the hip of the standing leg.*

*A very strengthening pose for the legs, core muscles and back.*

*Extend one arm forward to work balance. Extend both arms forward to challenge strength, stability and alignment.*

# TRIANG VIRABHADRASANA VARIATIONS

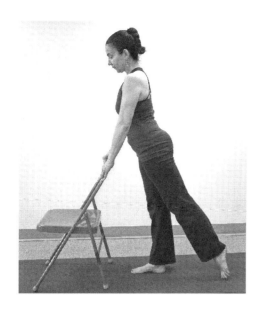 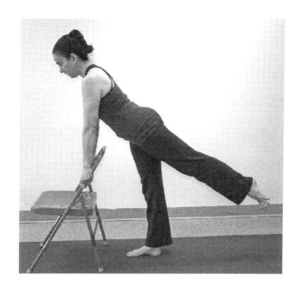

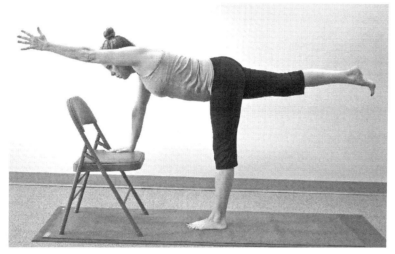

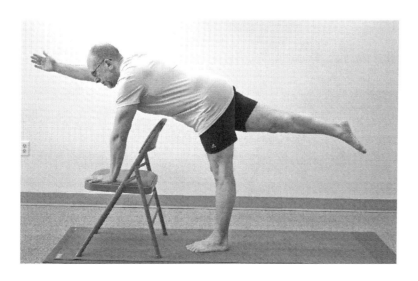

# PARSVAKONASANA
## Side Angle Pose

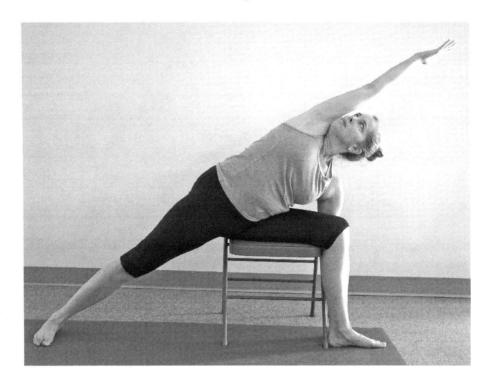

1. Sit the left thigh onto the chair seat, knee against the edge and extend the right leg out to the side.
2. Hips align to the long edge of the mat.
3. Arms extend out to the sides aligning with the shoulders.
4. Ground the base of the left big toe, little toe, outer heel to align the knee.
5. Ground the base of the right big toe, inner heel to outer heel to align the hips.
6. Extend the left arm and bring the hand to the outside of the left foot.
7. Bring the right arm along the side of the head and gaze up to the fingers.
8. Hold for 5 breaths, then repeat on other side.

**PROPS**

*If the chair seat is too low place a folded blanket or cushion under the thigh and adjust for individual stretch.*

*If the chair seat is too high place a block under the front foot to provide lift and proper alignment.*

*Rest the left forearm on the left thigh and extend the right arm.*

*Follow Parsva Virabadrasana with Utthita Parsvakonasana.*

# PARSVAKONASANA VARIATIONS

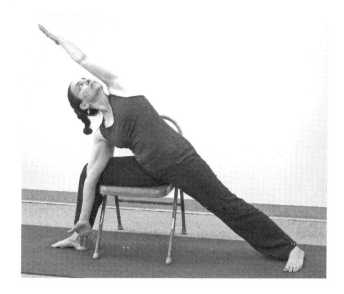

**NOTES**

*Feel free to flow from one warrior pose to the next placing one hand in front of foot or going deeper into a twist.*

*Be careful not to force the upper body in the revolves. Instead use the resistance of hand/arm to chair placement to hold the body in the pose.*

*In Parivritta Parsvakonasana the foot can be grounded or the heel lifted. This is an extreme stretch and should be held for 5 breaths.*

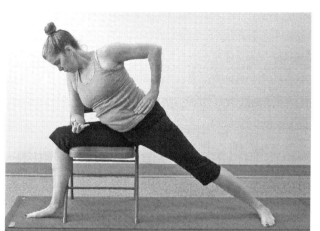

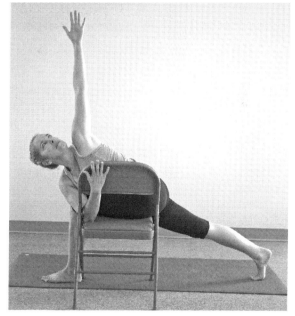

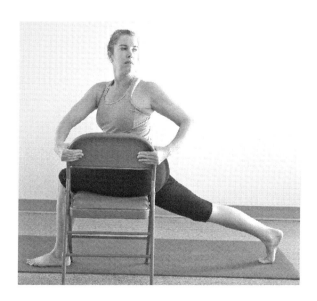

# PARSVOTTANASANA
## Intense Side Stretch Pose

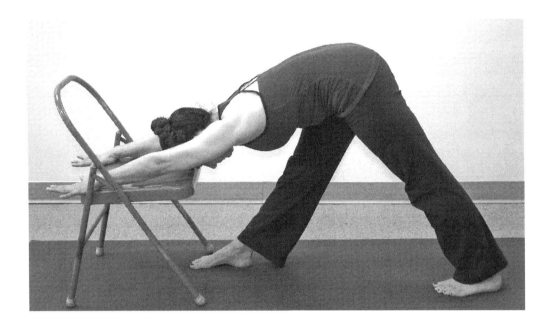

1. Come to standing pose (Tadasana) in front of chair seat with hands on hips.
2. Step right foot back and align feet to hip width.
3. Adjust body weight evenly between feet. Lift the belly, lengthen the spine and gaze forward.
4. Extend forward with a flat back, bringing the right hip back and left hip forward to align with each other.
5. Extend arms and place hands on chair seat lengthening the spine while keeping both legs straight.
6. Slowly move the chair forward away from the body increasing the stretch or stay and hold the pose for 5 breaths.
7. Come up slowly step forward and repeat on other side.

**NOTES**

*It is important to align the position of the legs and feet on two separate planes for maximum stability.*

*The objective is to extend the spine and broaden across the sacrum.*

*Hands can extend down to the chair legs or to the floor.*

*Sequence this pose with Parivritta Trikonasana (Revolving Triangle), or move into Surya Namaskar (Sun Salutation).*

# PARSVOTTANASANA VARIATIONS

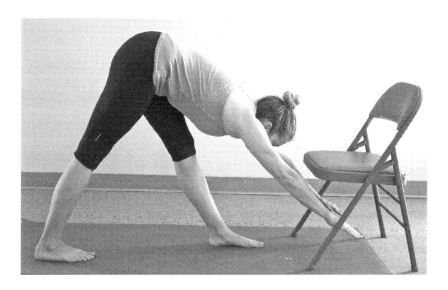

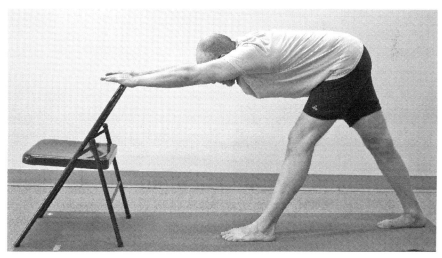

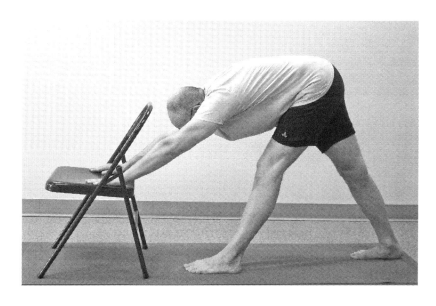

# PRASARITA PADDOTANASANA
## Feet Spread Intense Stretch Pose

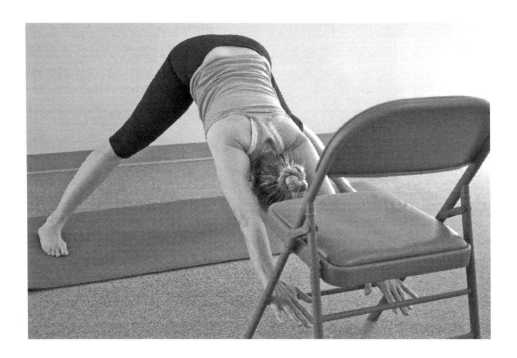

1. Step feet wide apart and place hands on hips.
2. Lifting from the hip bones to the rib crest and from the pubis to the base of the throat look up towards the ceiling.
3. Slowly come forward with a flat back and place both hands on chair seat.
4. Hold the pose for several breaths at each stage before lowering the hands.
5. Maintain full engagement of the four corners of the feet with the back of the legs aligned over the heels.
6. Hold for 5 breaths.
7. Lift the hands onto chair seat gently and come up to standing.

**NOTES**

*Following the extension bring hands to chair seat sequencing into Cat & Dog pose before returning to Tadasana.*

*The forehead can rest on the arms crossed on the chair seat.*

*This extension is similar to a wide legged Downward Facing Dog pose.*

*When in full extension lower the hands to the floor and walk them back to take hold of the ankles.*

# PRASARITA PADDOTANASANA VARIATIONS

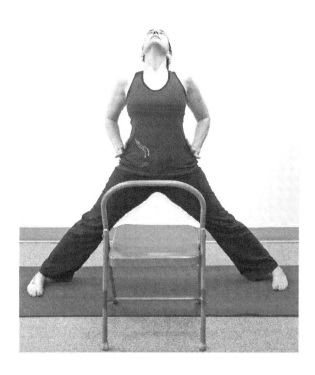
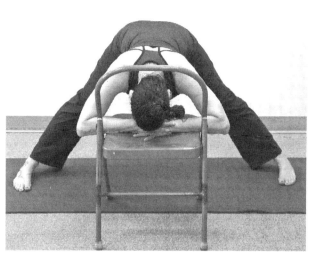
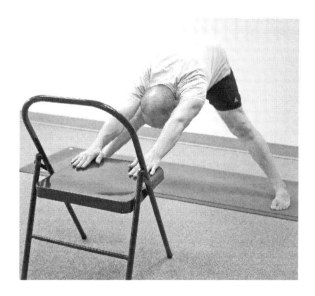
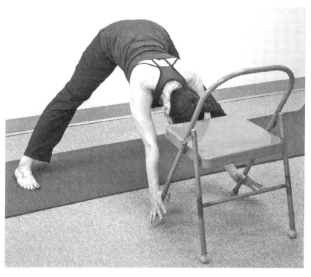

# NOTES

# BALANCING POSES

Vrikshasana
Urdhva Janu Sirsasana
Vasisthasana
Parsva Padangusthasana
Ardha Chandrasana
Natarajasana

Balancing poses using the chair allow for stability and maintaining proper alignment while holding a pose. Think of using the chair the way a ballet dancer works with the ballet barre.

Ballet class begins at the barre to properly warm, stretch and strengthen muscles and tendons, before stepping into the center of the room to perform sequences of dance combinations.

The chair can act as the yoga barre providing a stable object in which to stay steady and balance on one leg as the other extends, crosses or wraps.

In this sequence of poses there are variations on basic postures suited for first time novice and advanced students. They allow time to shift and adapt the body to the demands of a difficult asana.

Use blankets or folded mats to cushion the body and have an instructor or fellow student available to assist and correct.

# VRKSHASANA
## Tree Pose

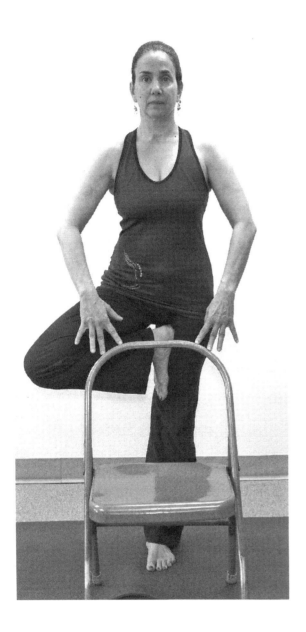

1. Facing the back of the chair rest the hands lightly on the upper edge.
2. Shift the weight to one leg and lift the other foot to the inner thigh of the standing leg. Toes should be facing the floor.
3. Align the right hip with the left.
4. Lift the space from hip bone to the lower rib crest.
5. Gaze forward and hold for 5 breaths.

**NOTES**

*This is a great knee and leg strengthening pose, as well as a hip opener.*

*The lifted foot can rest*
*\* with ball of foot on the floor and heel to ankle.*
*\* with foot resting against the calf muscle.*

*Resist placing the foot against the inside of the knee so as not to put pressure on that area of the leg.*

*One arm can extend to the ceiling or both hands can be pressed together in Anjali mudra (prayer position).*

*Mind is quiet and gaze is within.*

*Like a tree the foot will move and the leg shift, but strength and alignment will maintain the balance.*

# VRKSHASANA VARIATIONS

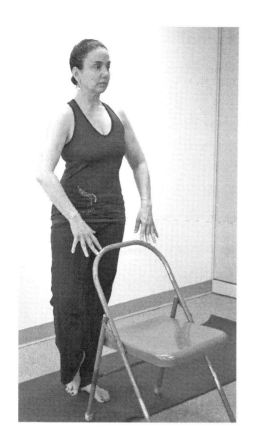
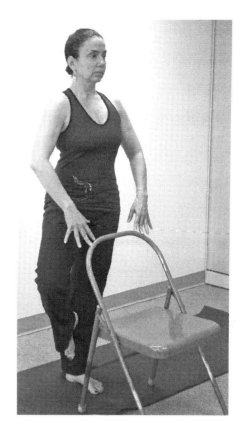

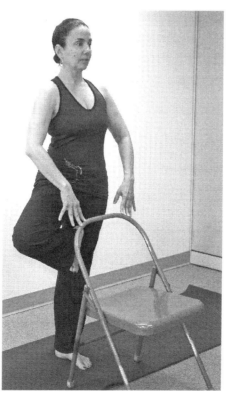

# URDHVA JANU SIRSASANA
## Standing Head to Knee Pose

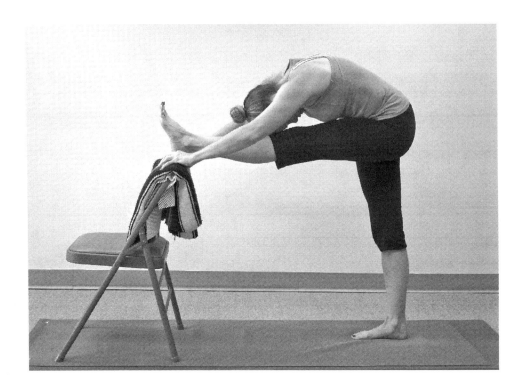

1. Place a blanket or folded mat on the back of the chair.
2. Place one heel onto the blanket and stand up straight, aligning the hips.
3. Standing leg is straight with foot facing forward. Ground the base of the big toe and outer heel.
4. Hinge forward from the hips placing the hands on either side of the extended foot and round the head towards the knee.
5. Keep eyes open and gaze to the floor.
6. Hold for 5 breaths.
7. Return to standing and extend arms out to the side revolving the upper body towards the extended leg.
8. Return to center and lift the leg from the chair and lower to the floor.

**NOTES**

*A revolving variation finds support with the chair while strengthening and preparing the body.*

*A simpler variation is to lower the arch of the foot to the chair back and bend the raised knee. This provides a deep stretch in the hip flexor on the standing leg.*

# URDHVA JANU SIRSASANA VARIATIONS

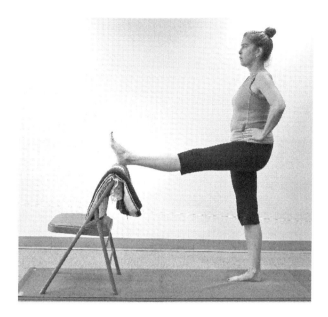

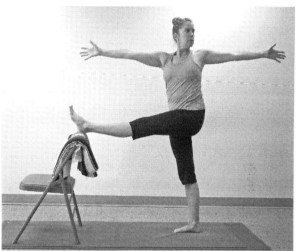

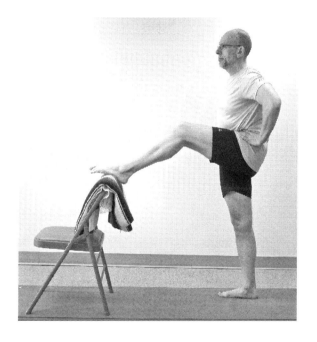

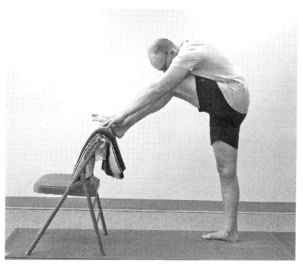

# VASISTHASANA
## Incline Pose

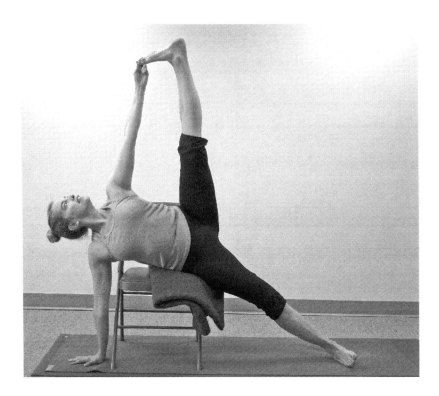

1. Place a blanket on the edge of the chair seat. Rest the right hip just above that edge.
2. Place the right hand on the floor, finger's pointing away from the chair.
3. Extend the right leg out with the edge of the foot on the floor.
4. Bend the left knee and bind the left index and middle finger to the big toe.
5. Extend the leg to the ceiling.
6. Bring the hips forward and the chest into alignment with the hips.
7. Gaze up to the foot. Hold for 5 breaths.
8. Lower the leg and repeat on the other side.

**NOTES**

*Maintain a slight lift, using the grounded hand and foot, so as not to be heavy on the seat.*

*Be careful not to hyper-extend the elbows. Align one shoulder over the other and one hip above the other.*

**PROPS**

*Place a block under the grounded hand to provide more lift.*

*Hold the pose with both legs together and arm along the side of the body or with arm extended to the ceiling.*

# VASISTHASANA VARIATIONS

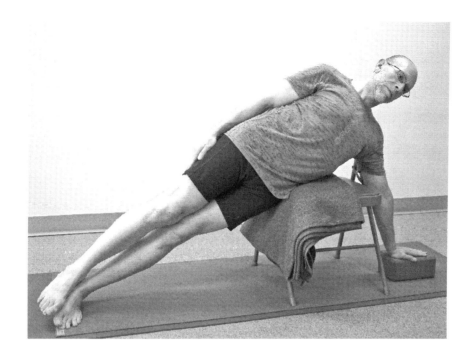

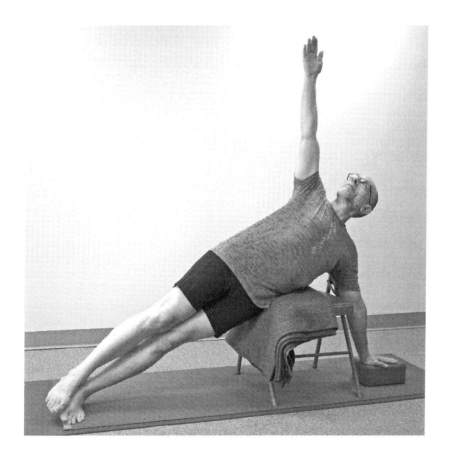

# PARSVA PADANGUSTHASANA
## Side Hand to Big Toe Pose

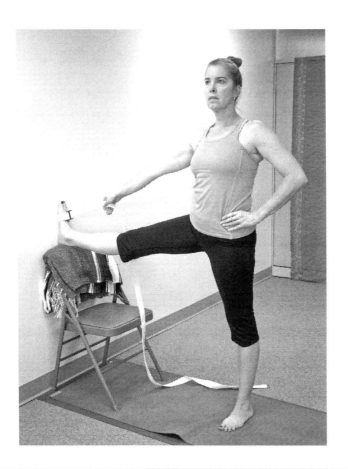

1. Place the chair back against the wall with a blanket or folded mat over the top edge.
2. Stand with chair to the right side and lift the right foot onto the chair. Loop a strap around the foot and place the heel of the right foot onto the blanket with the foot flat against the wall.
3. Hold the strap with the arm extended.
4. Gaze forward or to the left. Hold 5 breaths, then repeat on other side.

**NOTES**
*The foot flat against the wall provides stability while holding the pose.*

*Externally rotate the thigh of the extended leg keeping both hips in alignment with each other.*

**PROPS**
*You will need:*
*\* a folded blanket or mat*
*\* a strap*

# PARSVA PADANGUSTHASANA VARIATIONS

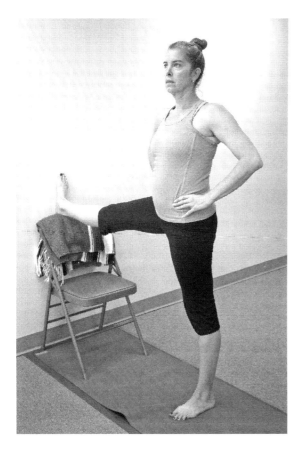

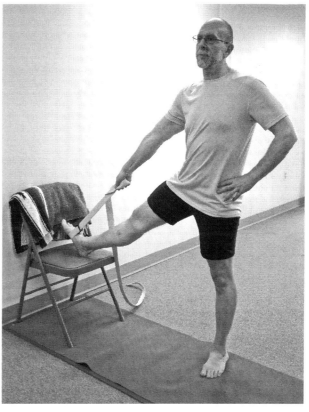

# ARDHA CHANDRASANA
## Half-Moon Pose

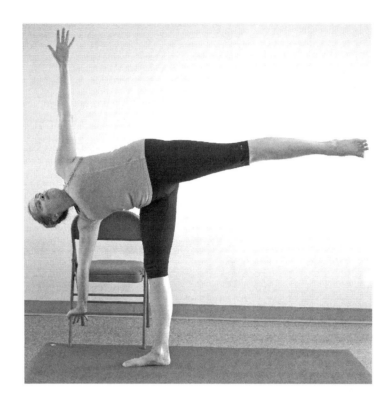

1. Prepare from either Parsva Virabadrasana or Parsvottansana.
2. With chair forward of the foot bend the right knee.
3. Reach right hand to low rung or leg of chair and lift left leg and straighten the right.
4. Take left hand behind to the chair back. Use for balance and to open the chest.
5. Rotate the chest and hip open and extend the left leg out and up, careful not to let it go behind the body.
6. Keep weight and stability on the standing leg and extend the left arm towards the ceiling.
7. Take gaze to the left hand and hold for 5 breaths. Bend the knee and return to Parsva Virabadrasana (Side Warrior).

**NOTES**

*Notice the placement of the chair before going into the pose. Make sure it is forward and to the side to allow for opening the body to the side.*

*Advanced variation: reach back and bind to the inside of the extended foot. Bend the knee and extend the leg up and behind the body. Chest and shoulders roll open and gaze is upwards.*

# ARDHA CHANDRASANA VARIATIONS

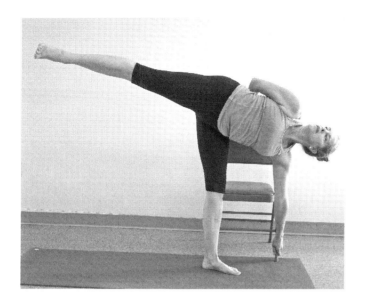

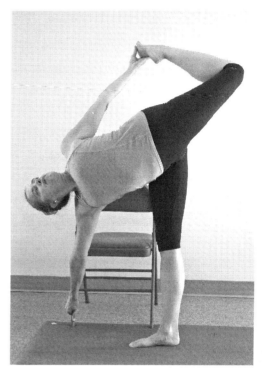

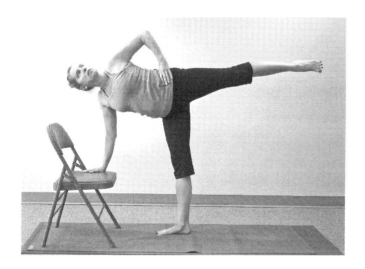

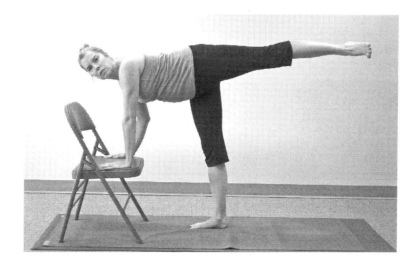

# NATARAJASANA
## King Dancer Pose

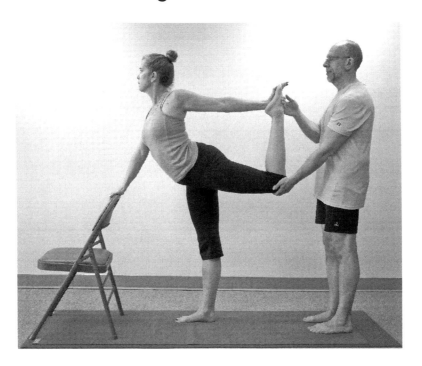

1. Stand between two chairs backs facing each other.
2. Place a blanket on one chair back.
3. Holding the chair in front bend the right knee, reach back with the right hand and lift the leg up onto the back of the chair.
4. Have an assistant hold the bent leg in place, align the hips and hold the pose.

5. Another variation is to face the wall and place one hand extended up the wall.
6. Standing leg is straight and weight is on the standing leg.
7. Hold for 5 breaths.
8. Come out of the pose slowly and repeat on other side.

**NOTES**

Natarajasana with the chair is best done with the assistance of the instructor or fellow student to help support the coming into, holding and coming out of the pose.

The chair should be the proper height for the student to rest the knee. If chair back is too high use a lower bench.

Be careful not to hyper-extend the standing leg by shifting all the weight onto the lifted bent knee.

This is a back bending pose as well, so lift up through the rib cage, broaden the shoulders and gaze forward.

# NATARAJASANA VARIATIONS

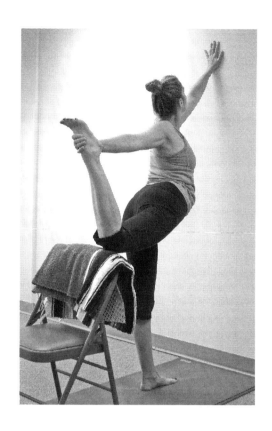
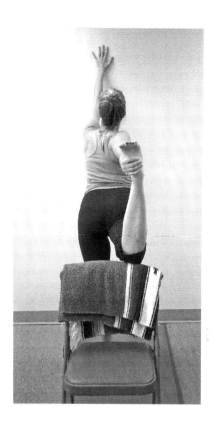

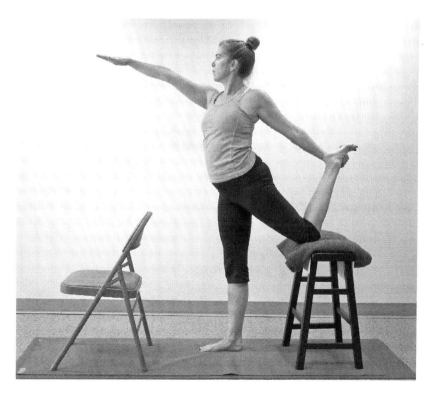

# SEATED POSES

Utkatasana
Salamba Eka Padasana
Garudasana
Pascimottanasana
Janu Sirsasana
Paragasana
Ardha Virasana
Upavishta Konasana
Baddha Konasana
Navasana
Balasana
Ubhaya Padangusthasana
Kurmasana

Seated poses are ideal for individuals who find standing poses difficult or tiring. Notice in the first chapter how standing poses can be done sitting on the chair. This allows for more of a flow from one posture to another without having to interrupt the focus on movement to breath.

This selection of seated poses can be combined for a vinyasa flow or added to sun salutations, balancing and floor poses.

Follow the seated poses with twists and revolving poses in the chair for a smooth vinyasa sequence.

Take your time, and remember the least amount of muscular effort for the maximum results is effortless effort.

# UTKATASANA
## Chair Pose

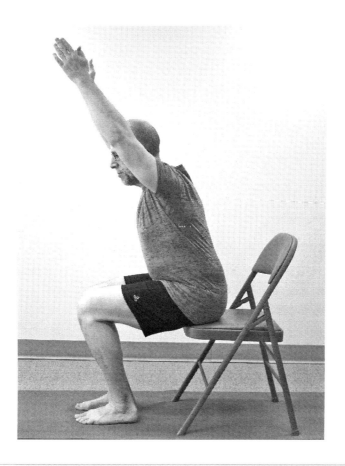

1. Sit forward on chair seat. Align the toes under the knees.
2. Feet forward, back straight and gaze ahead.
3. On the inhale lift the arms towards the ceiling and align them slightly forward of the ears.
4. Hold for 5 breaths. Shift weight to the feet and lift up off the chair.
5. Hold and slowly straighten to a standing position lowering the arms to the sides.
6. Inhale arms arise and slowly lower through chair pose back to sitting on the chair.
7. Repeat 4-6 times.

**NOTES**
*The lifting up off the chair and lowering back down to sitting is an excellent way to strengthen the legs.*

# SALAMBA EKA PADASANA
## Supported One Leg Pose

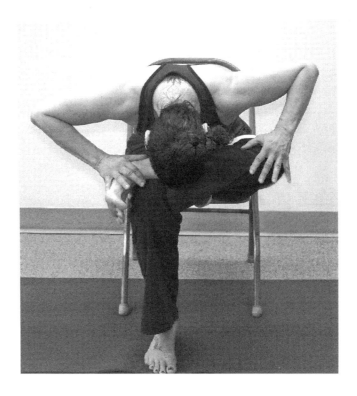

1. Sit center on the chair and bring the left knee into the chest. Lift elbows out to the side and broaden the upper back and chest.
2. Place the left ankle above the right knee on the thigh.
3. Place right hand on the ankle and left hand on the knee without pressing.
4. Roll forward and over the leg using the weight of the body to go deeper into the stretch.
5. Extend the hands down to the floor or back to the chair legs as a next step.
6. Hold for 5 breaths then repeat on other side.

**NOTES**

*This is a wonderful hip stretch. Be aware of the knee being careful not to push or force it downwards.*

*One variation is to cross the ankle further past the thigh or stay in Garudasana (Eagle pose).*

*Keep the elbows lifted out to the side when bringing the knee up to the chest.*

*Follow this pose with a seated Padagustasana (Hand to big toe pose, as shown in Sequences).*

# SALAMBA EKA PADASANA VARIATIONS

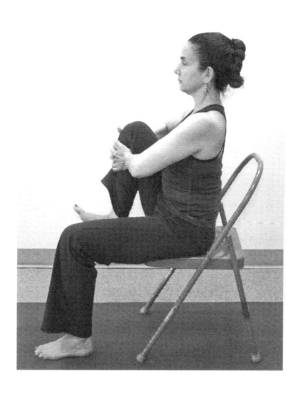

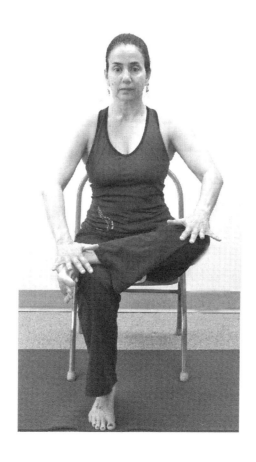

# GARUDASANA
## Eagle Pose

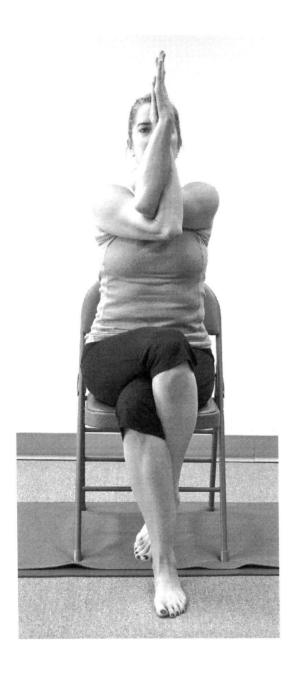

1. Sit forward towards the front edge of the seat.
2. Move the left foot center and cross the right leg over the left, wrapping the right behind the left, if possible.
3. Extend arms out to the sides and cross the right under the left in a big hug.
4. Take the right arm to the inside of the left elbow and the left to the outside of the right hand. Bring palms together if possible.
5. Gaze to the thumbs.
6. Hold here for 5 breaths.
7. Slowly come out of the pose and repeat on the other side.

**NOTES**

*If unable to wrap the top leg allow it to cross over and hang free.*

*If arms cannot bind hook one elbow inside the other or bring the elbows and inner arms together.*

*Before unwrapping the legs extend the arms out to the side and follow with a gentle twist.*

# GARUDASANA VARIATIONS

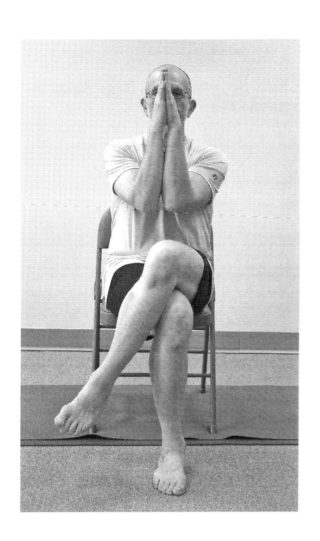

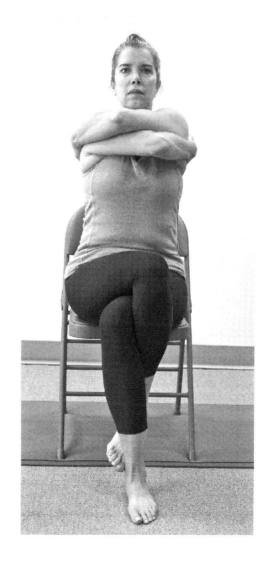

# PASCIMOTTANASANA
## Western Intense Stretch

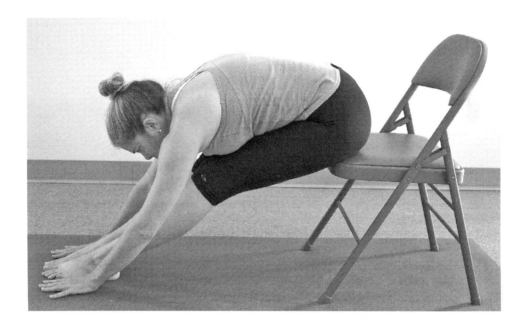

**Method 1**
1. Sit to the front edge of the chair. Extend legs out and ground the feet.
2. Extend forward lengthening the spine and bring the hands to the floor on either side of the feet.
3. Gaze to the toes, shoulders back from the ears and back extended. Hold for 5 breaths.

**Method 2**
1. Align two chairs of same height. Sit on one and place both legs on the other.
2. Extend forward taking the upper edge of the opposite chair.
3. Maintain a long, flat back, shoulders back from the ears and gaze forward to the toes.
4. Lower hands to the feet or chair for a more challenging extension.

*NOTES*

*This is a way to do Pascimottanasana for students having difficulty hinging forward from the hips when sitting on the floor.*

*It is important to maintain length in the spine so keep the arms high on the chair and lower as the body adjusts and opens to the stretch.*

*PROPS*

*Use a blanket under the hips to provide enough lift to support coming forward.*

*Place a blanket on the chair seat to cushion the forehead as it rests on the edge.*

*Prop the balls of the feet against the far rung of the chair to support foot and leg alignment.*

# PASCIMOTTANASANA VARIATIONS
## On and Off the Chair

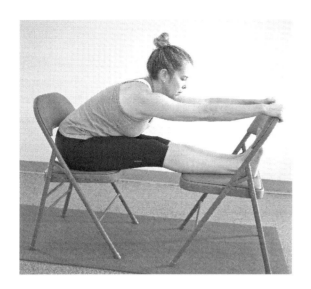
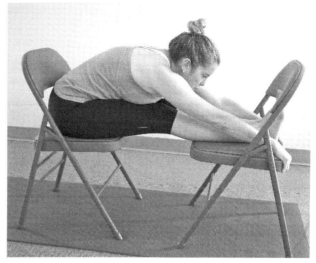
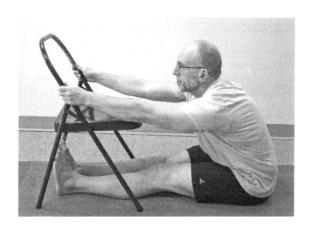
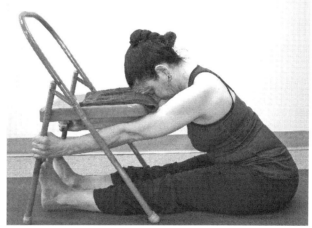
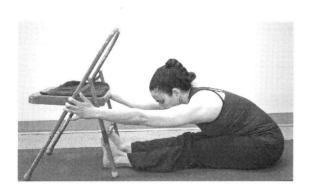
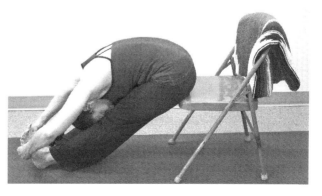

# JANU SIRSASANA
## Head to Knee Pose

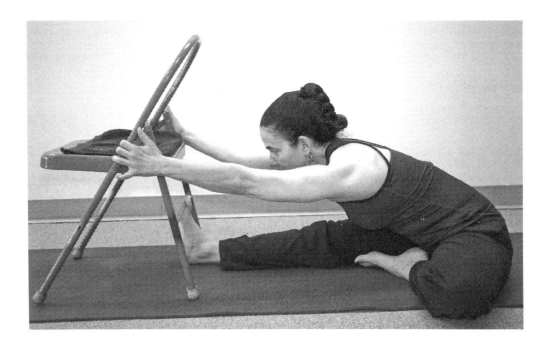

1. Sit on the floor and face either the front or the back of the chair.
2. Extend the right leg forward and bring the left foot to rest against the inside of the right thigh.
3. Place the ball of the right foot against the rung of the chair.
4. Take hold high on the chair to allow for lift and extension in the back and rib cage.
5. Gaze to the toes.
6. Lower the arms as the body adjusts and move deeper into the stretch. Hold for 5 breaths.
7. Come out of the pose and repeat on the other side.

**NOTES**

*For individuals with tight hips this pose can be done sitting forward on the chair with one leg extended and the other bent. Extend the upper body to the foot.*

*The more advanced version of Janu Sirsasana includes a rotation of the spine keeping the hips grounded and length in the vertebra.*

**PROPS**

*Place a folded blanket or wedge underneath the extended leg to keep from rolling over to the side.*

# JANU SIRSASANA VARIATIONS

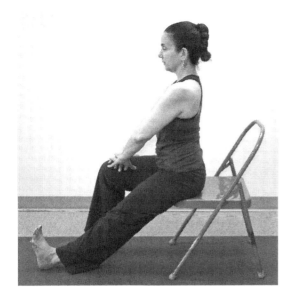
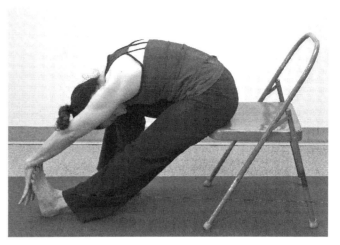

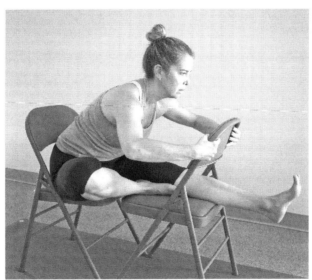

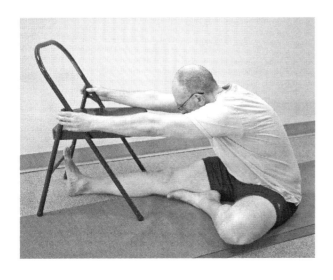
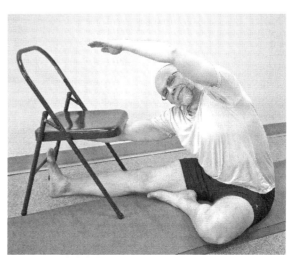

# PARAGASANA
## Closing the Gate Pose

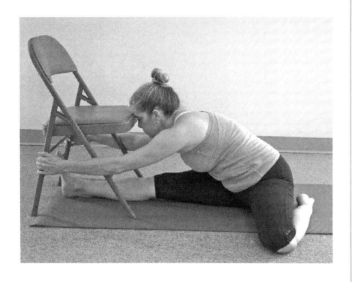

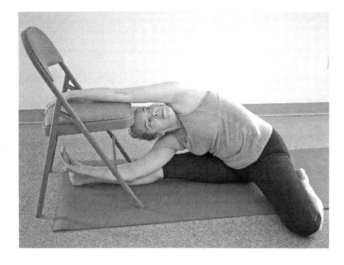

1. Sit on the floor facing the front of the chair seat.
2. Extend the right leg forward and bend the left gently aligning the knee to a 90 degree angle to the side.
3. The top of the left foot is on the floor directly behind the left buttocks. Ground the top of the big and little toes.
4. Lift up out of the hips and extend forward bringing the hands to the sides of the chair or lower as the stretch allows.
5. Rotate the right shoulder to the inside of the right knee. Extend and rotate the trunk of the body to follow the shoulder.
6. Take the right hand to the inside of the right foot and the left arm up and across the side of the head to the chair seat.
7. Hold for 5 breaths, then rotate back and over the right leg before coming up and changing legs.

### NOTES

*The rotation in Paragasana is similar to Janu Sirsasana. However, the bent knee's hip can lift up slightly off the floor. This allows for more revolve in the upper body.*

*The lower hand can take hold of the chair rung instead of the foot.*

### PROPS

*Place a yoga wedge or folded blanket under the hip of the extended leg to help maintain alignment.*

*A block can be placed under the extended leg's hip to provide lift to assist coming forward.*

# NOTES

# ARDHA VIRASANA
## Half-Hero Pose

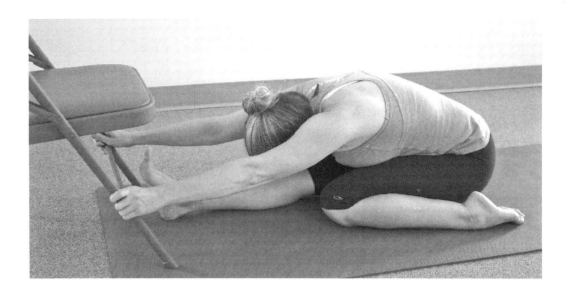

1. Sit on the floor facing the chair.
2. Extend the right leg and bend the left leg to the side. Keep the top of the foot to the floor.
3. Lift up out of the hips, hinge forward placing the hands on the seat or legs of the chair.
4. Keep both hips grounded to the floor and the extended leg straight if possible.
5. Gaze forward or to the knee. Hold for 5 breaths.
6. Extend the arms and lift up to a sitting position.
7. Change legs and repeat on the other side.

**NOTES**

*Keep the bent knee facing forward and in close to the opposite knee.*

*Ground the top of the big and little toe to the floor.*

*Lengthen forward from the hips rather than rounding from the back.*

**PROPS**

*Place a yoga wedge or folded blanket under the extended thigh and hip to provide stability and alignment.*

*Place a wedge or blanket under the buttocks to provide a slight lift to come forward.*

# ARDHA VIRASANA VARIATIONS

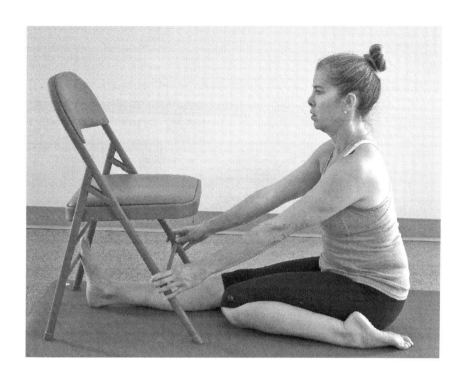

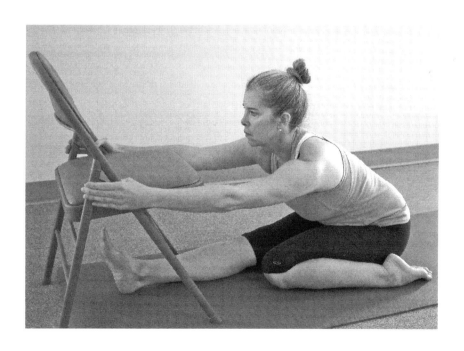

# UPAVISHTA KONASANA
## Seated Angle Pose

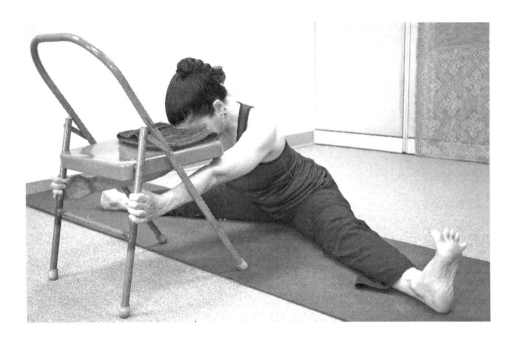

1. Sit on the floor facing the chair and open the legs out to the sides.
2. Lift the hips and extend the legs long then lower the hips back to the floor.
3. Tilt the pelvis forward and come forward bringing the hands to the chair.
4. Cross arms on chair seat and rest the forehead on the arms. Hold for 5 breaths.
5. Move the hands down the legs of the chair maintaining the extension in the back and the opening in the hips.
6. Hold another 5 breaths. Come up slowly and bring the legs together.

**NOTES**

*Come into this pose slowly and hold long enough for the adducting muscles to release and soften.*

*Individuals can sit upright and not come forward if flexibility in legs and back is limited.*

**PROPS**

*Place a folded blanket or yoga wedge under the buttocks bones to support the pelvic tilt forward.*

*Sit with the back to the chair using the edge of the seat to provide support for the lift in the spine.*

*Lean a bolster against the chair seat and rest the forehead against the bolster.*

# UPAVISHTA KONASANA VARIATIONS

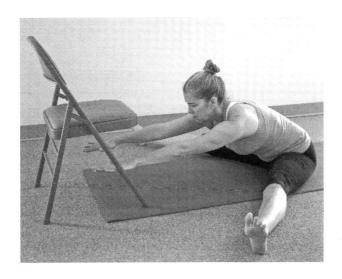

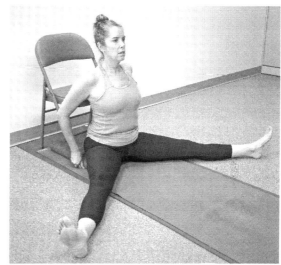

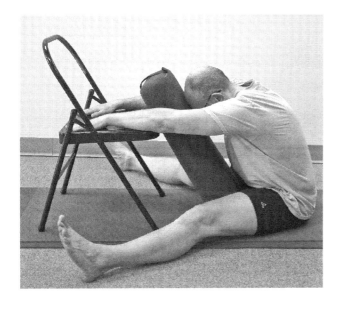

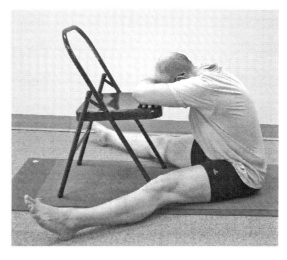

# BADDHA KONASANA
## Bound Angle Pose

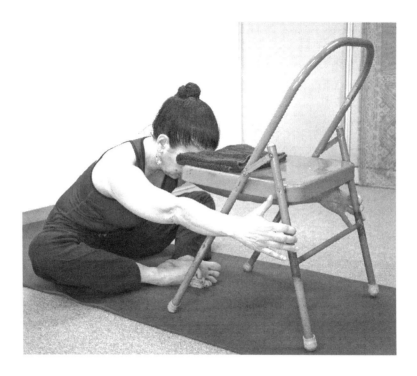

1. Sitting, face the front of the chair.
2. Bring the bottoms of the feet together and extend forward taking hold of the chair legs.
3. Rest the forehead on the front edge of the seat or fold the arms on the seat and rest the head on the forearms.
4. Feet can be forward to allow for more stretch or moved back towards the body if flexibility allows.
5. Keep an extended spine and soften the hips.
6. Use the exhale to release tension in the hips and move deeper into the pose. Hold for 5 breaths.

**NOTES**

*Variations include bringing two chairs together and sitting on one while bringing bottoms of the feet together.*

*With the bottoms of the feet together lower the hands between the chairs to the floor.*

**PROPS**

*Rest a bolster between the chair and hips and come forward to rest the head on the bolster.*

*Sitting on the folded edge of a blanket use the chair to lift the back and hold for 5 breaths before folding forward to the feet.*

# BADDHA KONASANA VARIATIONS

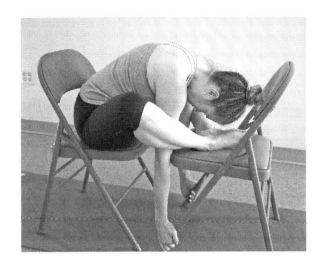 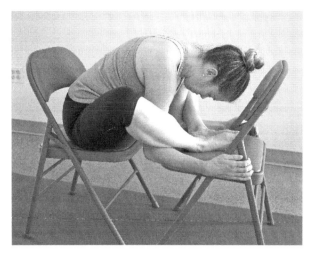

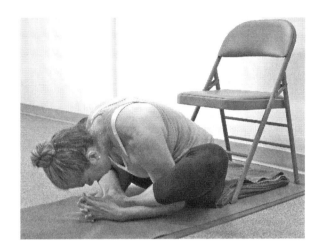 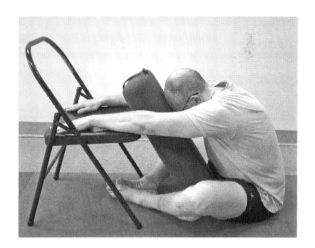

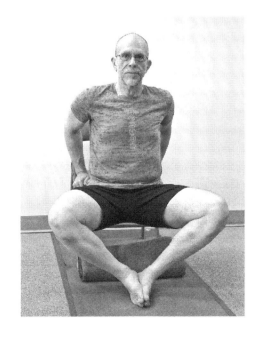 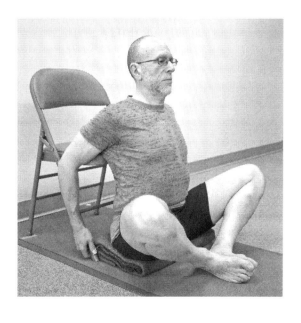

# NAVASANA
## Boat Pose

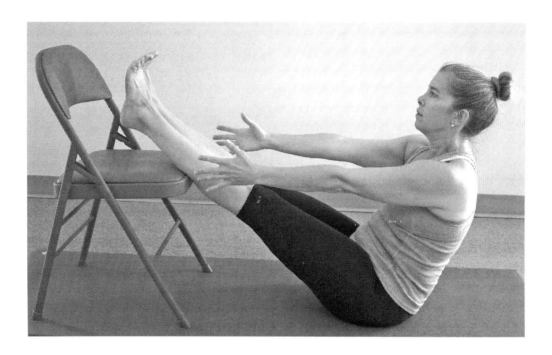

1. Sit on the floor facing the chair.
2. Prop the lower legs against the edge of the seat and straighten the legs.
3. Take hold of the edge of the seat with the fingers and lean back enough to engage the abdominal muscles, but not far enough to roll back to the floor.

4. Release the hands and extend the arms forward using a slight pressure with legs against the chair to maintain balance. Hold for 5 breaths.

**NOTES**

*Knees can be bent in Ardha Navasana resting the heels and calves on the chair seat.*

*Fingers can hook under the front edge of the seat while holding the pose.*

*Alternate lifting one leg and then the other before attempting to lift both together.*

*Keep the legs on the chair and roll the back down to the floor and tuck the chin and roll back up. Use this to strengthen the abdominal muscles.*

# NAVASANA VARIATIONS

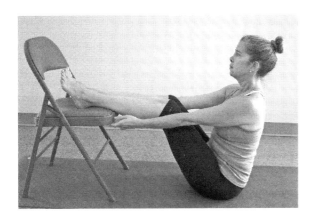
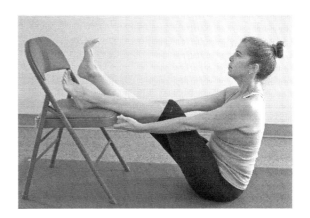

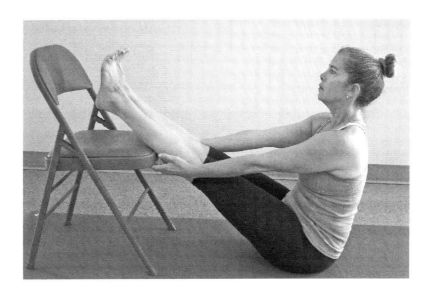

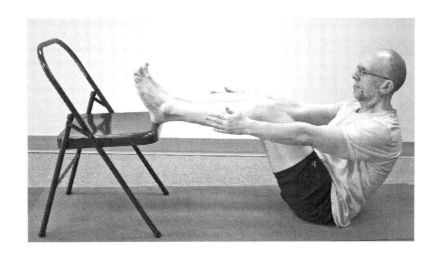

# BALASANA
## Child's Pose

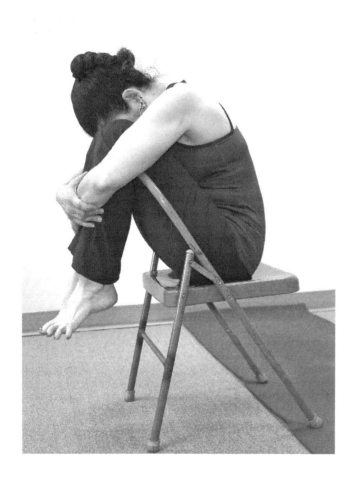

1. Sit on the chair and rotate around bringing your legs up and over the back rail of the chair.
2. Let the feet hang and round the upper body forward to the knees.
3. Wrap the arms around the legs or lower to the ankles.
4. Rest the head on the knees and hold for 5 breaths.

**NOTES**

*Use this pose to follow Ubhaya Padagustasana or precede it.*

*Sequence Balasana with the side twisting pose Bharadvajasana.*

*This variation of Child's pose works well for individuals who cannot kneel or sit on their heels.*

# UBHAYA PADANGUSTHASANA
## Both Feet Big Toe Pose

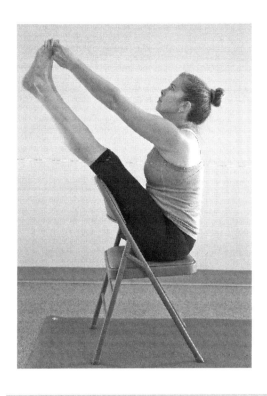 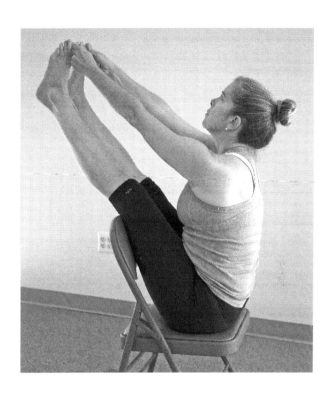

1. Sit on the chair facing the back rest.
2. Hook the index and middle fingers around the big toe and extend the legs up.
3. Keep the arms long, the back straight and the belly lifted. Gaze to the toes.
4. Use the back of chair as resistance for the legs to straighten.

5. Stay slightly forward on the chair and do not lean back too far.
6. Drop the shoulders down away from the ears. Hold for 5 breaths.
7. Release and fold the knees over the back of the chair and round forward into Balasana (Child's pose).

**NOTES**

*The abdominals come into play here and get a subtle strengthening from holding this pose.*

*Press the big toe against the fingers for a stronger connection.*

*Knees can be bent if difficult to extend fully.*

*Maintain an internal rotation to the legs.*

*A good variation for individuals who cannot extend their legs when sitting on the floor.*

# KURMASANA
## Tortoise Pose

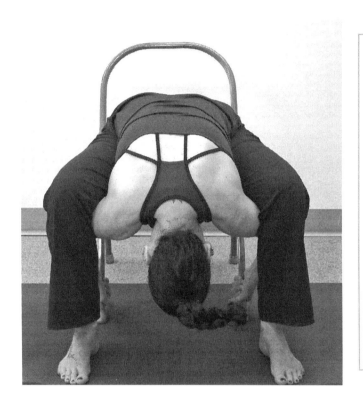

1. Sit forward on the front edge of the seat.
2. Open the legs wider than the hips with feet turned forward.
3. On the exhale roll down reaching the hands between the legs and to the legs of the chair.
4. Let the head hang naturally.
5. As flexibility increases take the hands up higher on the chair legs, even to the sides of the seat.
6. Keep the shoulders back from the ears and broaden across the upper back.

**NOTES**

*Variations of Kurmasana can include folding forward with knees wider and feet turned out.*

*Hands to the ankles on the outside of the knees.*

*A good preparation for Kurmasana on the floor.*

**PROPS**

*Place two blocks between and out in front of the feet and extend the hands forward before stretching back to the chair.*

*Place a bolster between two chairs and come forward to rest the torso along the length of the bolster.*

# KURMASANA VARIATIONS

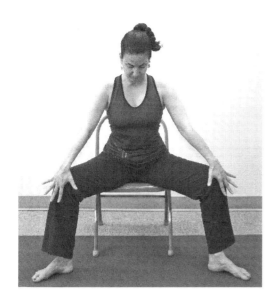
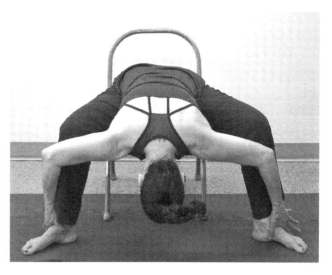

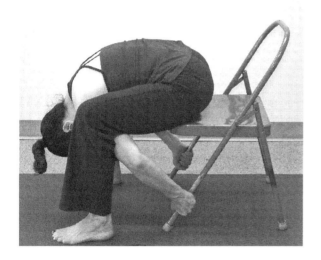
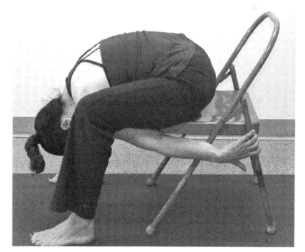

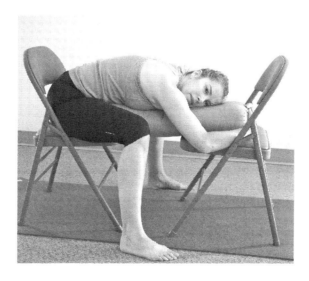

# BACK BENDING POSES

Urdhva Mukha Svanasana
Ustrasana
Shalabasana
Dhanurasana
Urdhva Dhanurasana
Eka Pada RajaKopadasana

Using the chair for back bending poses allows for a gradual and effective way to open the chest, stretch the intercostal muscles of the rib cage, and expand the heart and lungs.

Keep in mind that the major organs of the body are also muscles and will need time to stretch along with the rest of the body. This tightness and constriction can be caused by a diet high in processed foods and animal protein. A whole foods, low sugar, plant based diet will relax the organs, as well as, the entire muscular system creating more flexibility and ease of movement.

The chair can be used as a way to warm-up the back in preparation for self-supporting back bends and/or as a way to introduce back bending poses to beginner and intermediate students.

The support of the chair provides stability which allows the body to soften deeper into the pose without the fear of possible injury.

Be sure to prop the poses correctly with blankets and bolsters to support the back, neck and head.

# URDHVA MUKHA SVANASANA
## Upward Facing Dog Pose

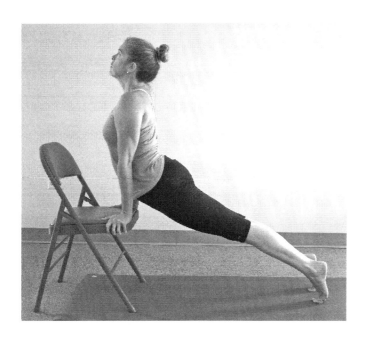

1. Turn the hands outwards on the front corner of the seat and come into a plank position.
2. Align the shoulders over the wrists and engage the legs with knees straight.
3. On the inhale lower the hips, open the chest and lift the spine; at the same time lifting forward onto the toes.
4. Lower the shoulders down from the ears, lift up from the belly, roll the biceps outwards and the inner elbow slightly inwards.
5. Gaze is forward or up to where the ceiling meets the wall. Hold for 5 breaths.
6. Flow out of Upward Facing Dog back into Downward Facing Dog.

### NOTES

*Variations can include facing the back of the chair with the hands on the top edge and turned out to the sides.*

*This is a backbend and is best served by bringing the hips towards the chair and using the strength of the arms to lift and open the upper body.*

# USTRASANA
## Camel Pose

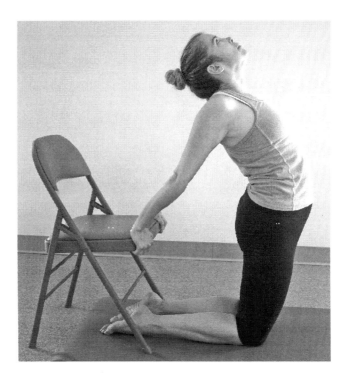

1. Kneel on the floor in front of the chair seat. Align the heels just under the front edge.
2. Inhale and lift, open the chest and reach back to place hands on the front edge of the chair.
3. Keep the thighs coming forward, the shoulders roll open and gaze is to the ceiling.
4. Lengthen the tailbone towards the floor to avoid pushing into the lower back. Hold for 5 breaths.
5. Come out of the pose and sit on the heels in Vajrasana.
6. Follow with a gentle twist or into Balasana, Child's pose.

**NOTES**

*Place thighs against the wall and upper edge of chair back just below shoulder blades. Extend the arms down the side of the chair legs as the chest lifts and opens.*

*Sitting in Vajrasana with toes tucked lay back onto the chair aligning the front seat edge just below the shoulder blades.*

*Sitting in Vajrasana lay back onto the chair aligning the front seat edge just above the shoulder blades.*

*Variations for Ustrasana include a deeper back bend, by reaching the hands overhead to the chair.*

# USTRASANA VARIATIONS

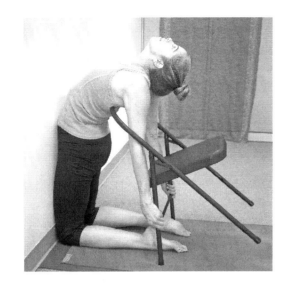
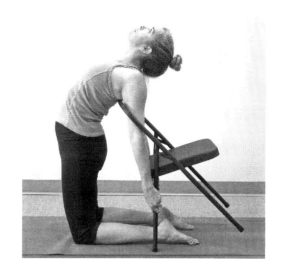
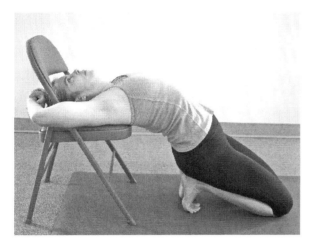
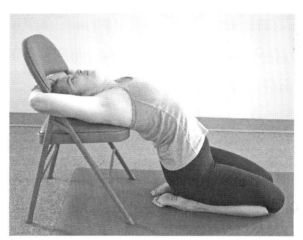
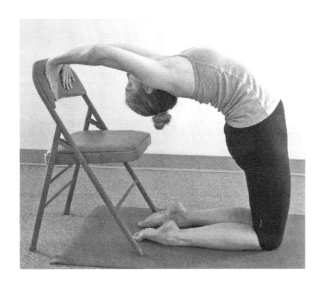
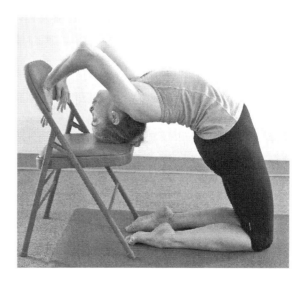

# SHALABASANA
## Locust Pose

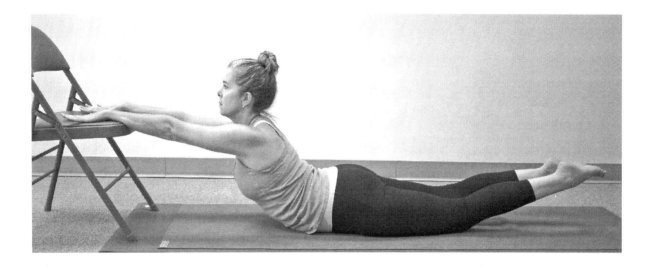

1. Lay on the belly with arms extended forward towards the chair.
2. Begin by lifting the upper body and placing the hands on the first rung or the chair legs.
3. Hold 5 breaths and lower down.
4. Turn the head and rest a moment.

5. Repeat the first pose and this time lift the feet and legs a few inches off the floor. Hold, release and rest.
6. Inhale and lift the upper body and legs placing the hands on top of the chair seat. Hold 5 breaths, release and rest.
7. Flow into Balasana or Adho Mukha Savasana to stretch out the back.

**NOTES**

*The support a chair provides for this backbend is beneficial for individuals with lower back pain.*

*These variations are a good introduction for students who are unable to lift the upper body off the floor. Begin low and work up to the seat over time.*

*Legs are extended and feet close or together.*

*Feet can remain on the floor in the beginning and are lifted as the student progresses in strength and flexibility.*

# SHALABASANA VARIATIONS

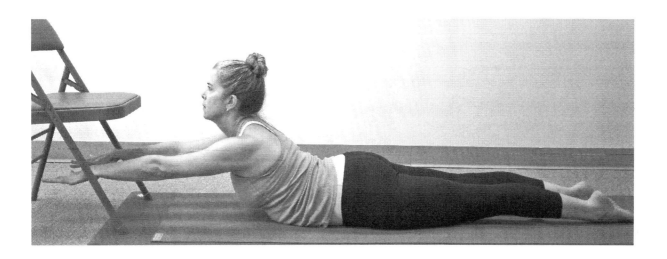

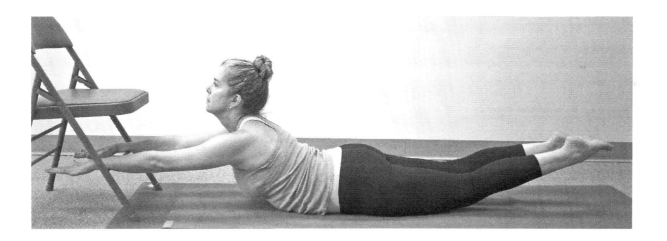

# DHANURASANA
## Bow Pose

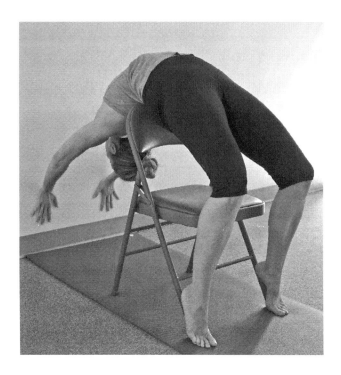

1. Face the back of the chair to the wall a good arms length from the chair.
2. Sit on the chair, back against the back rest. If needed place a folded blanket over the top edge of the chair back.
3. Rest the heels of the feet against the front legs of the chair with the balls of the feet grounded to the floor.
4. Take the arms behind and interlace the fingers. Extend the arms long and tuck the chin to the chest.
5. Rest the hands on the back legs of the chair and lift the hips up, laying the back onto the back edge and grounding the heels and balls of the feet.
6. Bring the hands out to the wall and extend the arms, walking the hands down the wall as flexibility allows. Hold for 5 breaths.
7. Come down slowly and follow with a twist then a forward bending pose.

**NOTES**
*It is important to keep the balls of the feet grounded to the floor and the heels pressing into the chair legs to maintain chair stability.*

*Hands can slide down the chair legs or remain on the the back edges of the chair seat.*

**PROPS**
*Fold a blanket and lay it over the upper back edge of the chair to cushion the spine.*

# DHANURASANA VARIATIONS

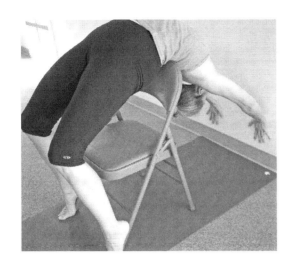

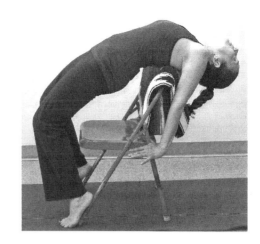

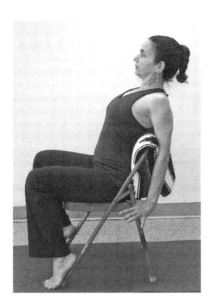

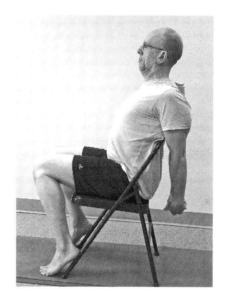

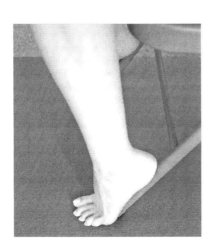

# DHANURASANA VARIATIONS

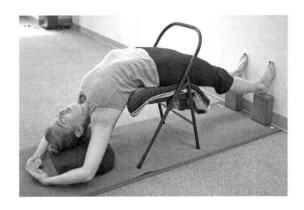 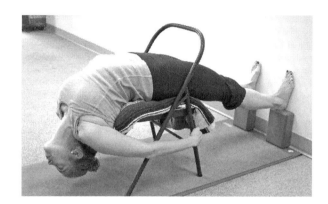

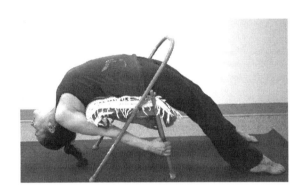 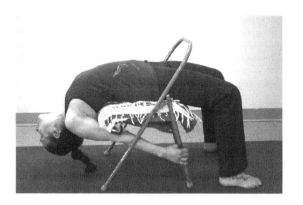

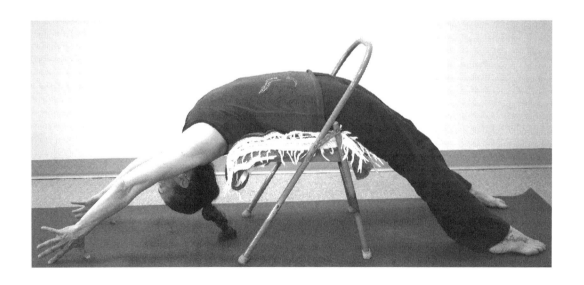

# URDHVA DHANURASANA
## Upward Bow Pose

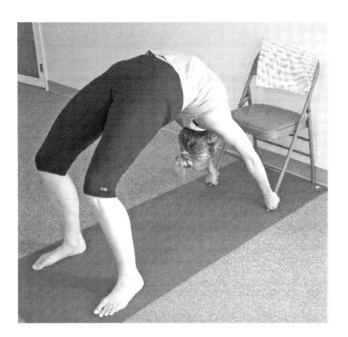

1. Place the chair against the wall and a blanket or rug pad along the back edge of chair.
2. Lay on the back, bend the knees and bring the feet in towards the buttocks.
3. Extend arms overhead and take hold of the lower front legs of the chair.
4. Press down with the hands, tilt the pelvis and lift the hips up off the floor.
5. Use the feet and legs to power the hips higher. Continue to press down onto the chair legs and lift upwards. Hold for 5 breaths.
6. Follow with a twisting pose.

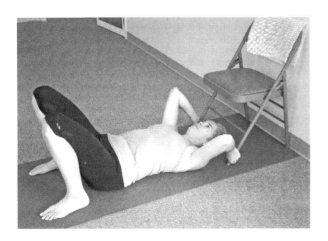

**NOTES**

*It is important to remember to push down with the hands rather than lift or pull away from the wall.*

*Stretch the legs to bring the shoulders over the wrists keeping the elbows straight and the chest open.*

*Ground the inner edge of the feet maintaining an internal rotation to the legs.*

# EKA PADA RAJAKAPOTASANA
## King Pigeon Pose

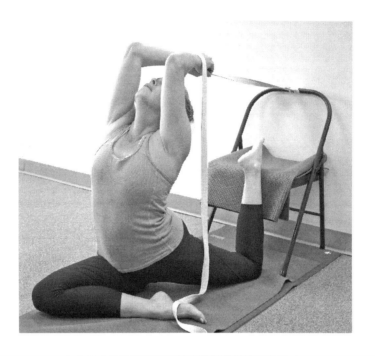

1. Place the chair against a wall. Loop a strap around the back edge of the chair. Cushion the chair seat with a folded mat or blanket.
2. Kneel on the floor, bend the right knee and bring the right heel in line with the left hip.
3. Bend the left knee and place the front ankle against the edge of the seat.
4. Extend the left arm back to the foot and take hold of the strap.
5. Carefully rotate the left elbow upwards and take hold with the right hand.
6. Press the chest forward and up, sit down into the pose and keep hips aligned.
7. The gaze can be forward or to the ceiling. Hold for 5 breaths.

**NOTES**

*The variations for King Pigeon help to prepare the body for a deeper stretch on the floor.*

*The bent leg on the chair seat stabilizes the pose and helps to position the hips.*

*In pigeon on the floor face the back of the chair holding to the upper edge to provide lift in the back bend.*

*The standing variation is a simple way to open the hips when flexibility is limited. If chair is too high stand on a solid block.*

# RAJA KOPADASANA VARIATIONS

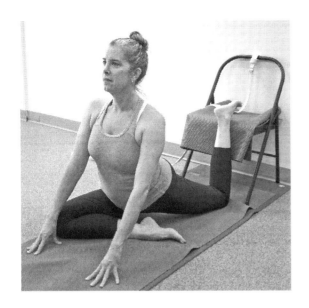
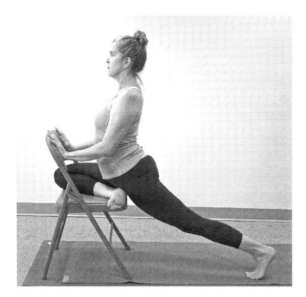

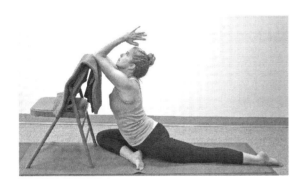
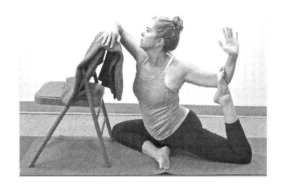

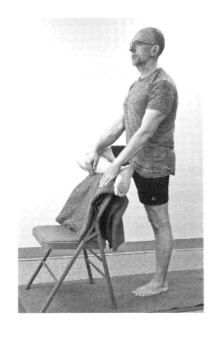
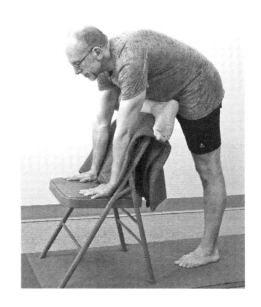

# TWISTS & REVOLVING POSES

Marichyasana
Ardha Matsyendrasana
Bharadvajasana
Pashasana
Utthita Marichyasana

Twisting poses with the chair are used to support the extension of the spine when turning. They can be done sitting on the chair or on the floor in front of the chair.

A **revolving pose** is a gentle rotation of the upper back with gaze over the shoulder. This is recommended for pregnant women, those with spinal limitations or before doing a full twist.

A **twist** asks more of the spine, taking the rotation deeper into the lower back.

There are many safe and gentle ways to twist and revolve the spine especially using the chair to stabilize the body.

Remember to keep the back lifted, the spine straight, both buttocks grounded and use the eyes to guide the neck into the rotation.

Never force or pull into the pose. Listen to the body and it will reveal how far it is willing and able to go.

# MARICHYASANA
## Great Sage Pose I

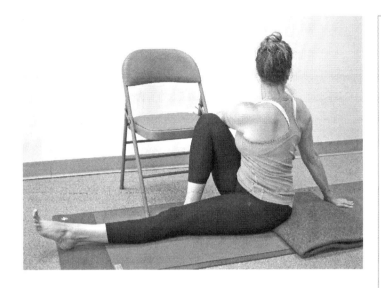

1. Sit on the floor on the edge of a folded blanket; with the chair to the side of the mat and seat forward.
2. Extend the left leg, bend the right knee, bring the foot to the side of left knee.
3. Support the right knee against the chair.
4. Inhale, lift up and begin to revolve to the right.
5. Extend the left arm over the right knee and take hold of the chair.
6. Bring the right hand to the floor behind right hip.
7. Take the gaze over the right shoulder. Hold for 5 breaths then change sides.

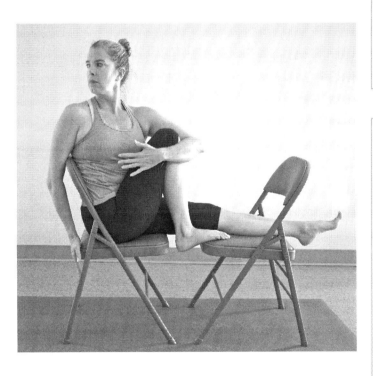

### NOTES

*This simple revolve focuses on the upper body turning while the pelvis is quiet and stable.*

*Variations include using two chairs and wrapping the opposite arm around the bent knee. This works for individuals who cannot get up and down off the floor.*

*Keep the extended leg internally rotated with toes toward the ceiling.*

# ARDHA MATSYENDRASANA
## Great Sage Pose II

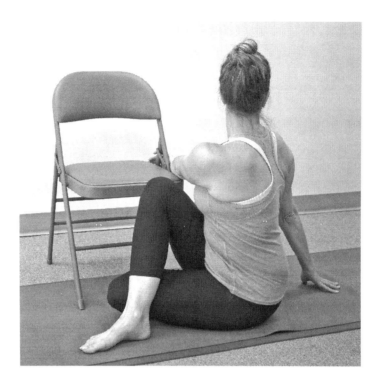

1. Sit on the floor with the legs extended forward.
2. Bend the left knee and bring the heel to the outside of the right buttocks.
3. Bend the right knee and cross the foot over the left thigh.
4. Keeping the buttocks on the floor raise the left arm and cross it over the right thigh.
5. Use the edge of the chair to keep the right knee aligned. Ground through the right foot.
6. Twist the torso using the gaze to look over the right shoulder.
7. Place the right hand behind and aligned with the right hip. Use it to help lift the back rather than push further into the twist.
8. Hold for 5 breaths.

**NOTES**

*Extend one leg with other knee bent and foot placed on the outside of the straight leg.*

*Use of two chairs for those who cannot go to the floor is a stable way to twist the spine.*

**PROPS**

*A folded blanket or yoga wedge placed just under the buttocks.*

# MATSYENDRASANA VARIATIONS

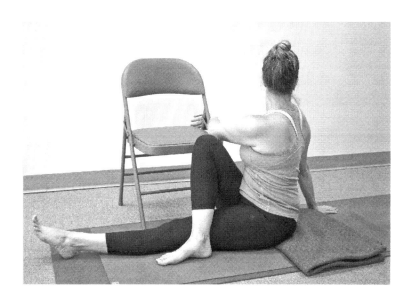

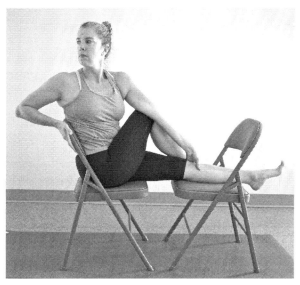

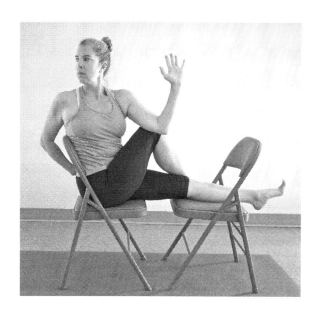

# BHARADVAJASANA
## Twisting Pose

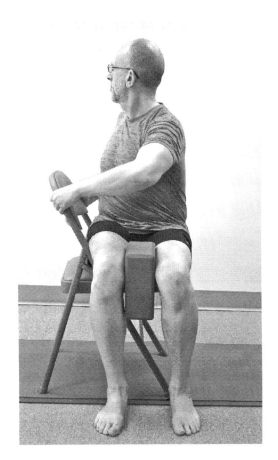

1. Sit on chair and place a block between the knees. Feet hip distance apart.
2. Lengthen the spine and turn towards the back of the chair with hands on opposite sides of the chair back. Keep elbows lifted and out to the sides.
3. Keep both hips grounded and gaze over the shoulder.
4. Hold for 5 breaths. Release and turn to the other side.

### NOTE
*Variation is to sit with legs through the back of the chair. This can follow deep back bending poses such as Dhanurasana.*

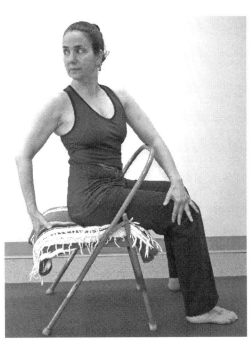

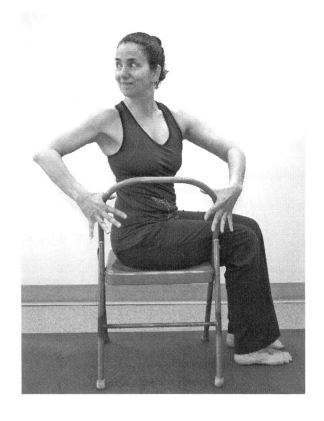

# PASHASANA
## Advanced Twisting Pose

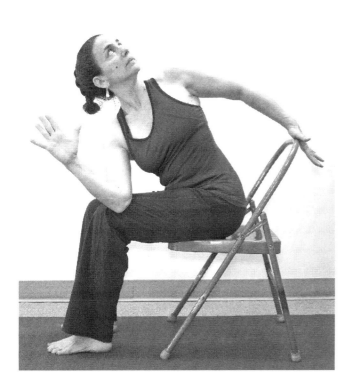

1. Sit on the chair with feet and legs together.
2. Twist to the left and bring the right elbow across the left thigh.
3. Reach back and take the left hand to the upper back of the chair.
4. Use the eyes to turn the neck and look back and up over the left shoulder.
5. Reach the right hand down the outside of the left thigh and bind to the chair leg.
6. Hold for 5 breaths.
7. Return to center before twisting to the other side.

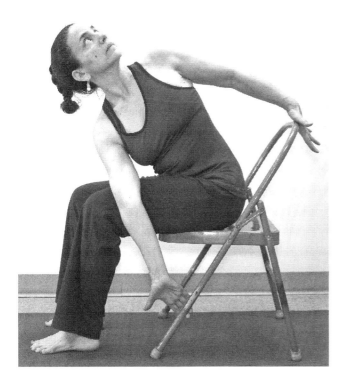

**NOTES**

*This is a nice preparation for more advanced floor twists and binding poses.*

*Listen to the body and do not force the back into an aggressive twist.*

*Keep both buttocks on the chair as the spine lengthens in the twist.*

# UTTHITA MARICHYASANA III
## Extreme Twist Pose

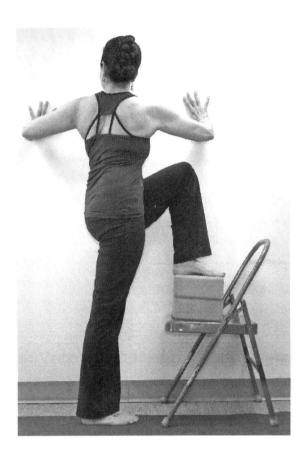

1. Place the chair next to the wall. Place 1-2 blocks on seat to position the knee higher than the hip.
2. Stand with left hip touching the wall.
3. Lift the left foot and place it on the blocks.
4. Place both hands on the wall, and revolve to the left with elbows bent, shoulder height and hip against the wall.
5. Use the gaze to turn the head and look over the left shoulder.
6. Hold for 5 breaths.
7. Return to center and lower the leg.
8. Repeat on the other side.

**NOTES**

*Place foot on the chair seat if unable to lift the foot higher.*

*Maintain the hip against the wall while twisting.*

*This twisting variation is for individuals who find it difficult to rotate the spine from a sitting position, as well as for releasing tension in the lower back.*

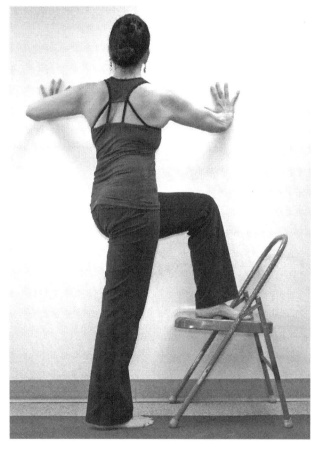

# INVERSIONS

Bujan Dhanurasana
Halasana
Sarvangasana
Pincha Mayurasana
Salamba Sirsasana
Adho Mukha Vrkshasana
Savasana

Going upside down can be a daunting experience for students in the beginning of their practice. Use the chair to learn poses and strengthen in preparation for self-supported inversions. This helps to minimize any fear or anxiety.

Always prop students with folded blankets under the shoulders to avoid placing too much pressure on the neck.

Make sure to set students up properly and observe how they move into and out of the pose. Not only do they have to invert their body but they have to maneuver the chair as well.

Have plenty of blankets, bolsters and blocks on hand to assist and support the poses.

Most of all teach inversions with a sense of fun and enjoyment. Going upside down is what your students did as children and the memories of youthful spontaneity comes from how you as the teacher approach the asana.

# BUJAN DHANURASANA
## Shoulder Bow Pose

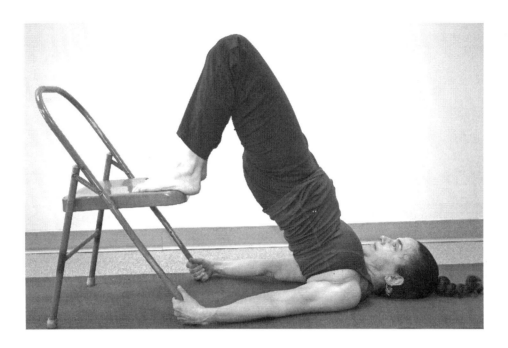

1. Lay on the floor feet facing the front of the chair seat.
2. Place the arch of the feet on the front edge of the seat and take hold of the two front legs of the chair.
3. Slowly lift the hips coming to rest on the shoulders. Maintain the weight in the shoulders and off the neck.
4. Chin is tucked but not so much to cut off the breath. If necessary lift the chin slightly.
5. Hold for 5 breaths.
6. Come down or flow into a variation of walking one leg at a time overhead into Halasana (Plow pose), and back again to the chair.

**NOTES**

*Variations with this pose can include extending one leg to the ceiling then lower and repeat with the other leg.*

*Hands can come to the lower back for more support and lift to the spine.*

**PROPS**

*Place a folded blanket under the shoulders as in Halasana to prevent excess pressure on the neck.*

*See the Sequence chapter for flow variation using Bujan Danurasana.*

# BUJAN DHANURASANA VARIATIONS

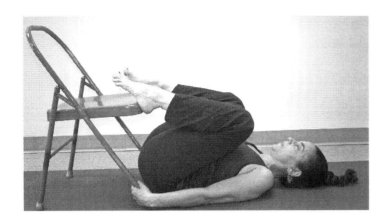

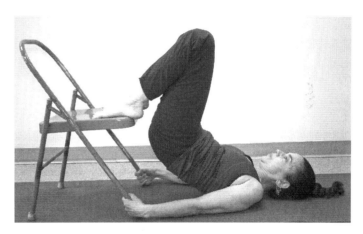

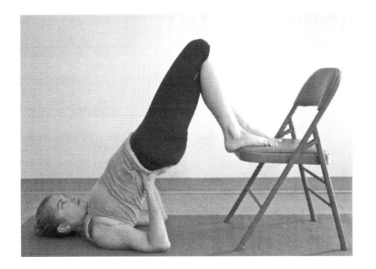

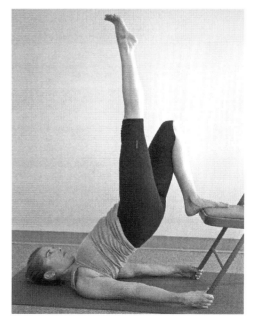

# HALASANA
## Plow Pose

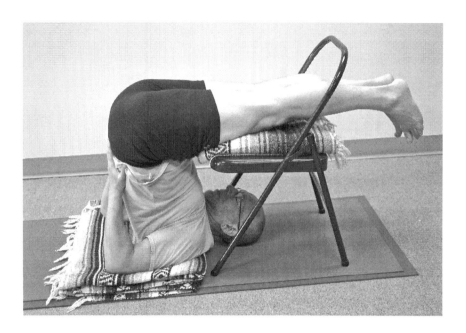

1. Lay on the floor with the head under the front edge of the chair seat.
2. Bend the knees and lift the hips up and overhead bringing the legs onto the seat, the legs extended through the back.
3. Make subtle adjustments as needed.
4. Bring the hands to the lower back for support and lift, keeping the elbows in towards each other.
5. Hold for 1-5 minutes.
6. Roll down out of the pose slowly and rest before proceeding.

**NOTES**

*With the thighs on the chair seat this becomes a resting pose and can be held for up to 5 minutes.*

*Variations include moving the chair to leg length and resting only the toes on the chair.*

*Hand and arm positions can vary in their placement.*

**PROPS**

*Place 1-3 folded blankets under the shoulders to better support the neck. Shoulders rest on the edge of the blankets.*

*The fold of the blanket is directly under the shoulders.*

*Place a folded blanket on the chair to cushion the legs or provide height.*

# HALASANA VARIATIONS

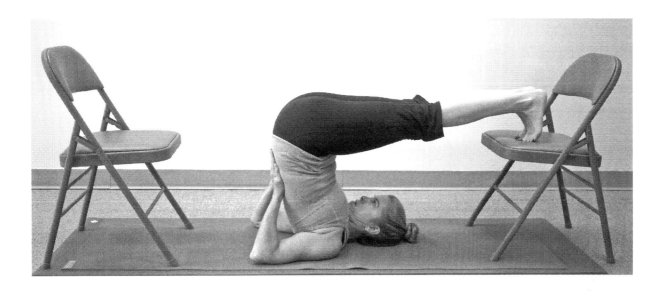

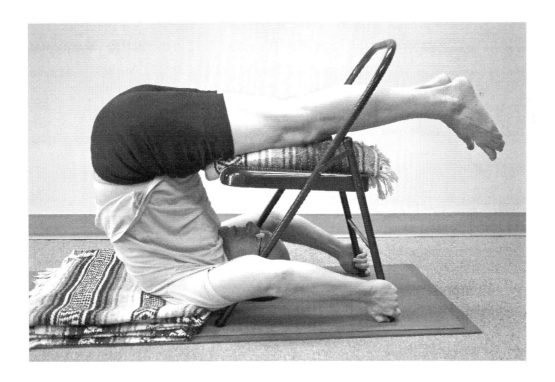

# SARVANGASANA
## Shoulder Stand

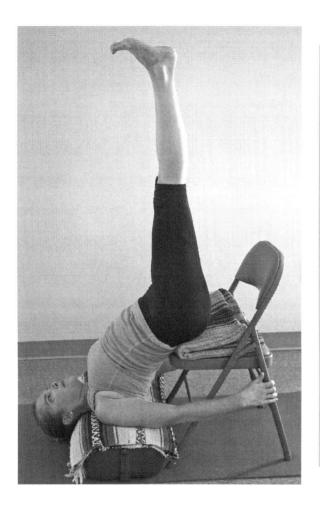

1. Place a folded blanket on the seat of the chair to cushion the front edge.
2. Place a bolster on the floor in front of the chair and cover with 1-2 blankets depending on the length of the torso.
3. Sit on the chair facing the back and hook the legs over the back edge.
4. Take hold of the chair sides and lower down slowly until the shoulders rest on the far edge of the bolster and the sacrum (lower back) rests on the seat edge.
5. Extend both legs towards the ceiling maintaining an internal rotation. Activate the feet in Pada Bandha (foot lock) to keep the legs dynamically charged.
6. Hold up to 5 minutes or longer.
7. To come out of the pose lower the legs over the back back and use legs and hands to pull up to sitting.

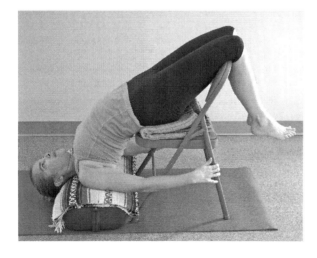

### NOTES

*This variation of shoulder stand can be used by individuals who have neck or shoulder issues.*

*The support of the chair and bolster promotes relaxation in the body-mind.*

*A good pose for expanding the lungs and opening the chest.*

# PINCHA MAYURASANA
## Peacock Pose

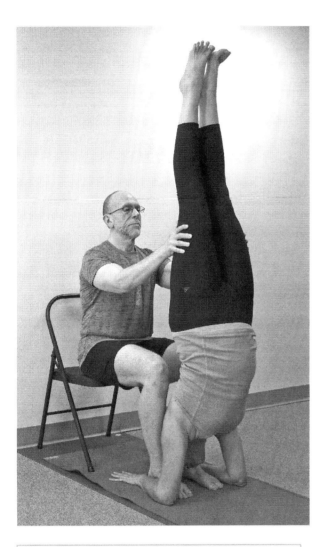

1. Have an assistant sit toward the edge of the chair seat.
2. Begin on all fours and lower the forearms to the floor aligning shoulders over elbows. The assistant's shin bones support the shoulders.
3. Lift the hips and walk the legs in towards the arms. Extend one leg and lift the weight onto the forearms, wrists, hands and fingers. The assistant supports the lift and helps maintain stability.
4. Gaze is to floor.
5. Hold for 5 breaths.
6. Return to the floor slowly and rest in Balasana (Child's pose).

**NOTES**

*A variation of this pose is with the back to chair seat lower forearms to the floor. Interlace the fingers, lift the hips and place the feet on the front edge of the chair. Align the shoulders over the elbows and hold for 5 breaths.*

*A great way to strengthen the upper body for self-supporting inversions.*

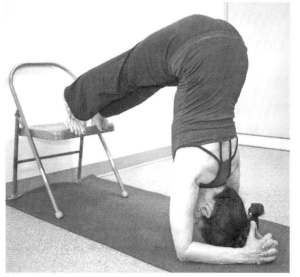

# SALAMBA SIRSASANA
## Supported Head Stand

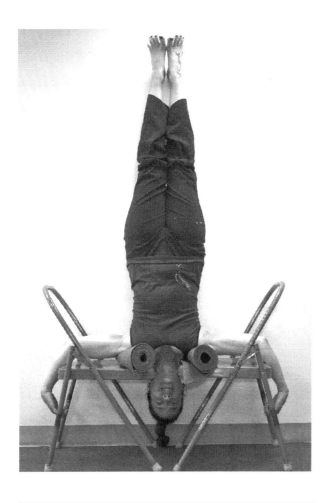

1. Place two chairs against the wall facing each other. Leave enough space to slide the neck through.
2. Place two rolled mats or folded blankets on the edge of each chair.
3. Step the legs out wider than the hips, fold forward and slide the neck between the chairs, resting the shoulders on the mats.
4. Extend the arms across the seat of the chairs.
5. Bring one knee and then the other onto the seat of each chair. Hold here and breathe.
6. Bring the knees into the chest, extend up straight and lean them against the wall. From here work on balancing without the wall for support.
7. Hook the fingers around the back chair rungs for support.
8. Stay lifted yet relaxed and settle into the shoulders allowing the head to hang naturally and the neck to extend.
9. Hold for up to 5 minutes.
10. To come down bend knees and bring them to rest again on the seat of the chairs. Place the feet on the floor and slide the head out, standing up slowly to acclimate the brain. Complete with Balasana (Child's pose).

### NOTES
*This variation works well for individuals who cannot go onto their heads due to head or neck issues.*

*Individuals receive the benefits of being upside down without having to place pressure on the head.*

### PROPS
*2 rolled mats or folded blankets.*

# SALAMBA SIRSASANA VARIATIONS

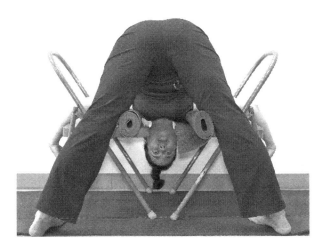

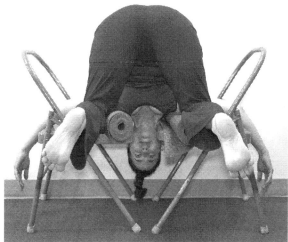

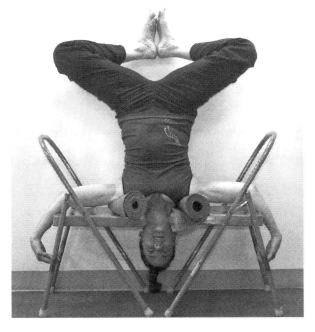

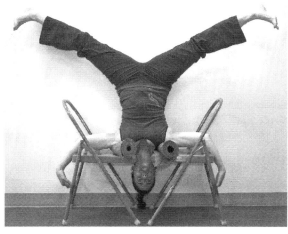

# ADHO MUKHA VRKSASANA
## Half Handstand Pose

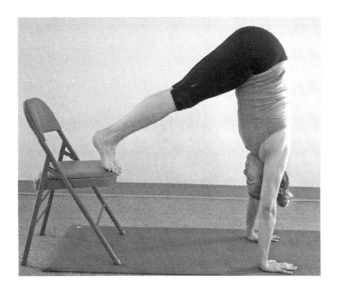

1. Place the chair at the back of the mat and come into downward facing dog pose.
2. Walk the hands about half way back to the feet. Lift one foot at a time onto the front edge of the chair seat.
3. Bring the hips up and align over the shoulders and wrists.
4. Allow the head to hang freely and bring the shoulders back from the ears.
5. Lengthen up through the spine to the tailbone.
6. Hold 5 or more breaths.
7. Come down and rest in child's pose.

**NOTES**

*This handstand variation can be incorporated into a vinyasa flow.*

*For building strength walk the hands out into a plank position leaving the feet on the chair. Do a few pushups or Chaturanga Dandasana then walk back to half handstand.*

*Extend one leg towards the ceiling, lower and extend the other.*

*Have an assistant support walking the legs into a full handstand.*

*Keep the heels lifted and the weight more towards the toes.*

*Remember to press down to lift up.*

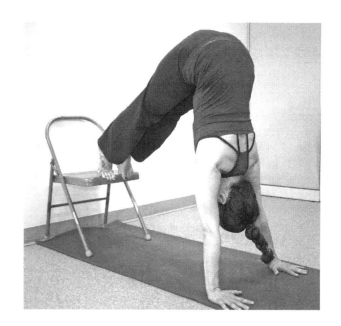

# SAVASANA
## Corpse Pose

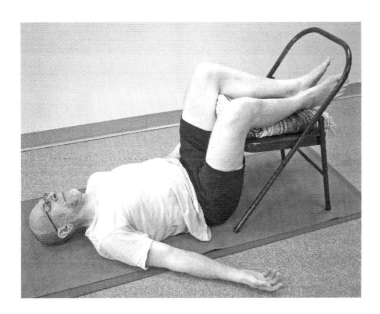

1. Sitting, face the chair and lay back onto the floor.
2. Place the legs onto the seat and bring the feet through the opening.
3. Scoot the hips forward to rest under the knees and let the legs relax and fall out to the sides.
4. Rest the arms on the floor, adjust the neck, soften the eyes, jaw, tongue and face.
5. Quiet the mind and rest for up to 20 minutes.

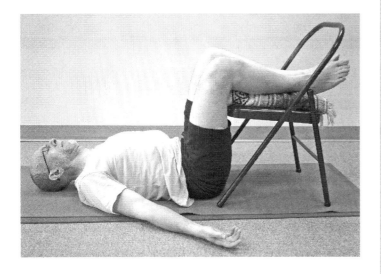

*NOTES*

*This variation of Savasana allows for a deep relaxation and is restorative to the legs.*

*Bringing the hips in under the knees allows the psoas muscle to soften and relax after working to keep you stable throughout the practice.*

*PROPS*

*Place a folded blanket under the legs to cushion and for more height as needed.*

# SEQUENCES

Simple Movements
Sun Salutation Sequence
Uttanasana Sequence
Cat & Dog Sequence
Sarvangasana-Halasana-Karnapindasana Sequence
Seated Warrior Sequences

At the heart of a Vinyasa Flow practice is the sequencing of poses moving in a way that supports the internal awareness of the body-mind.

Effortless effort means not to have to stop and start in a disruptive manner, but to move into, hold and move out of poses with smooth and stable transitions.

It takes time to learn all the poses and how they fit together in a flowing sequence, but the ones you will find in this chapter should help you understand how the poses and movements fit together.

Along the way, you will discover how to sequence favorite poses just by listening to the body's natural intelligence. Listen carefully and ask your body what it needs in the moment, then act on what you hear and know it to be true.

Never force, pull or act in an aggressive or harmful way. Instead, share the practice as if with a best friend and your body will respond in the most amazing ways.

## SIMPLE MOVEMENTS

Simple movements are gentle sequences to do before holding poses for a series of breaths. Opinions differ as to length of time one should hold a pose. One style may say 20 seconds and another count 5 breaths; there are those who listen to the body for how long to hold; and still another style calling for holding for 5-30 minutes.

Holding allows time for the pose to soften the limitations of the muscles and connective tissue that has the body bound up, stiff and inflexible.

These simple movements are used to awaken energy and focus the mind by bringing attention to the breath. Each inhale and exhale happens naturally as the length of the movement is matched to the length of the breath.

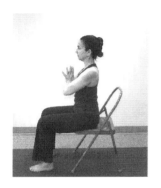 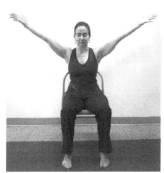 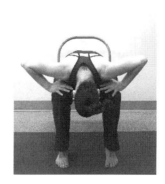 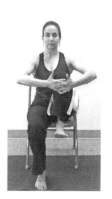

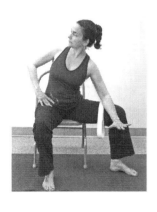 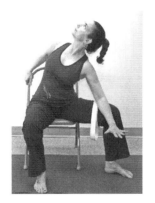 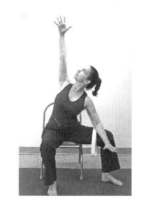 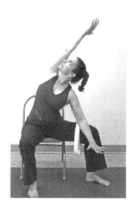

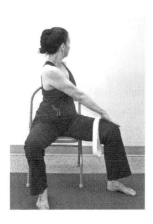 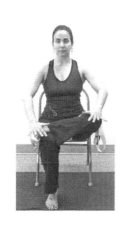 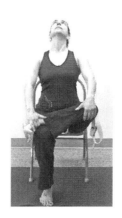 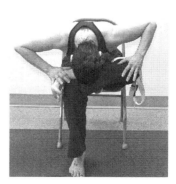

# SUN SALUTATIONS I

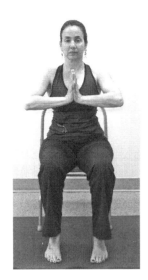 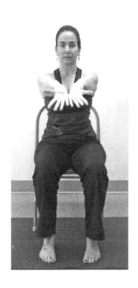 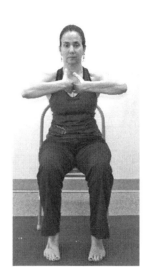 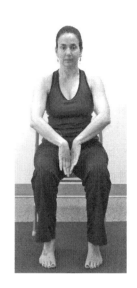

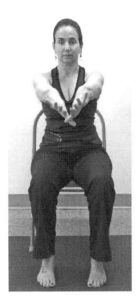 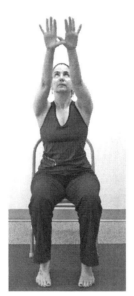 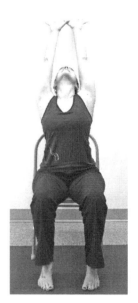

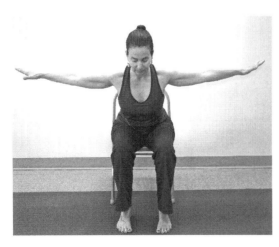 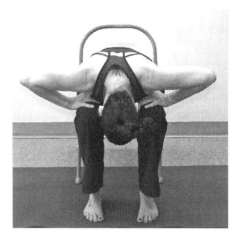

# SUN SALUTATIONS II

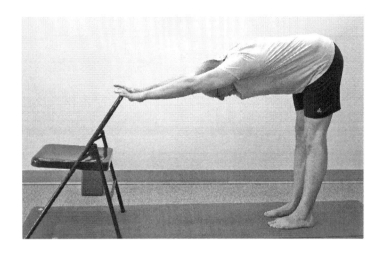

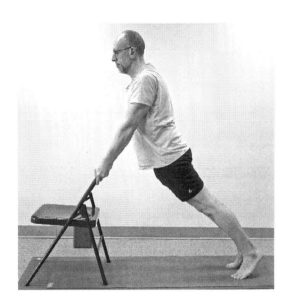

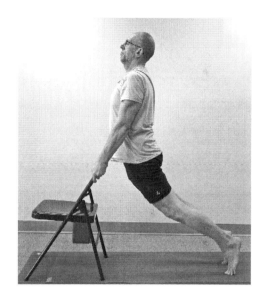

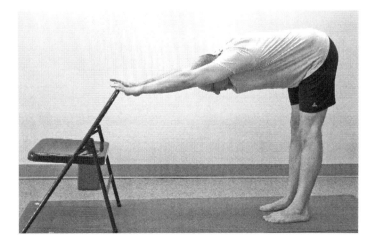

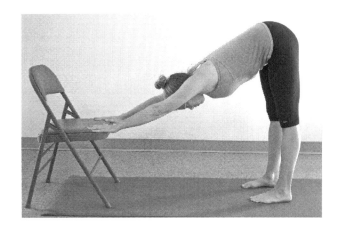
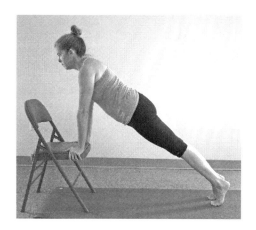

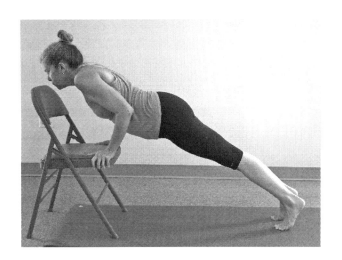
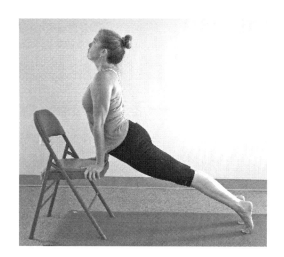

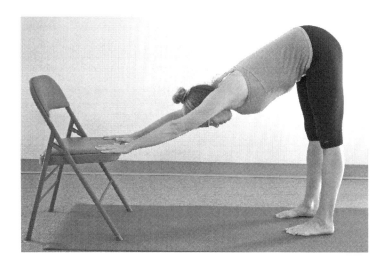

# UTTANASANA SEQUENCE

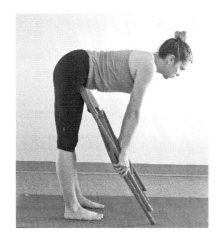 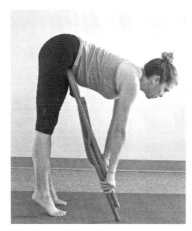 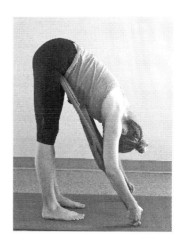

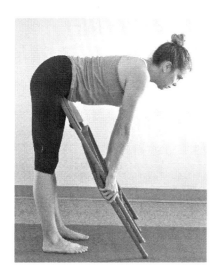 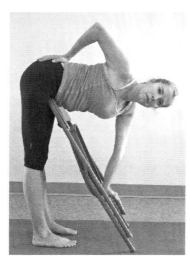 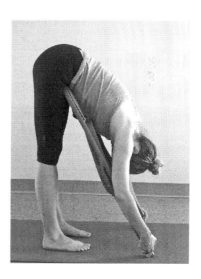

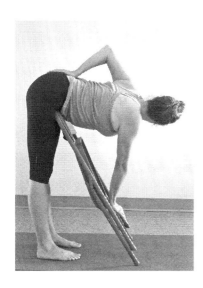 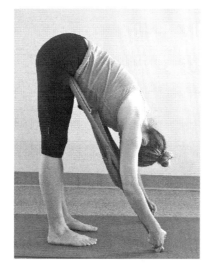 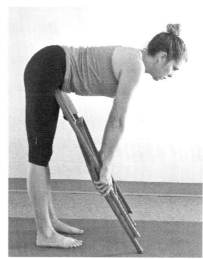

# SEATED CAT & DOG

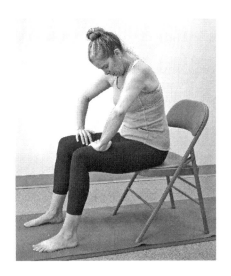 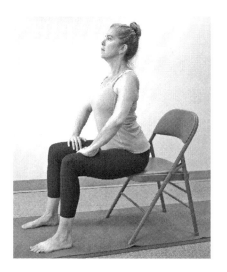

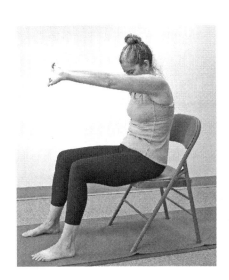 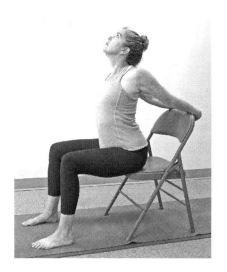

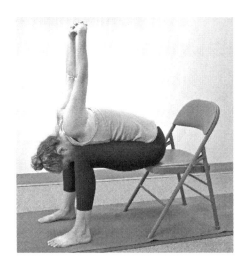

# SARVANGASANA-HALASANA-KARNAPINDASANA

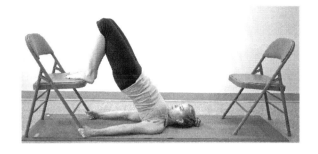 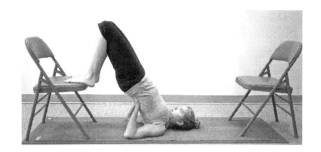

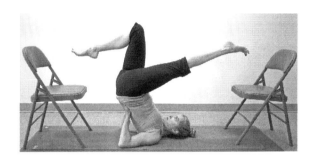 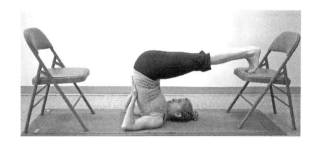

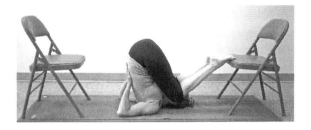 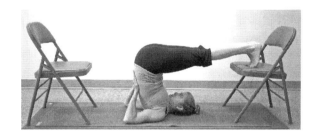

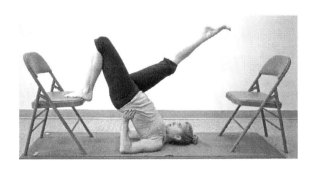 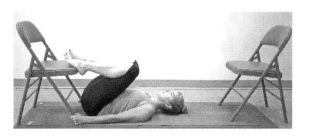

# ASANA SEQUENCES

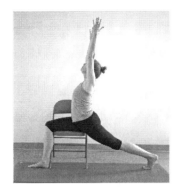 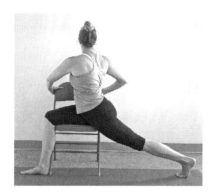 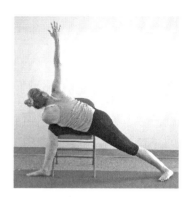

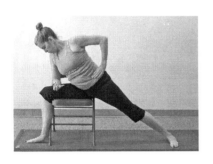 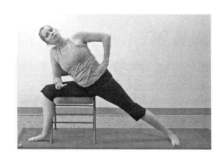 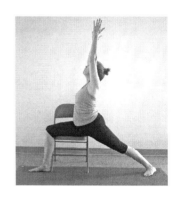

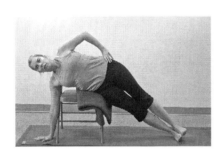 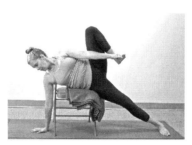 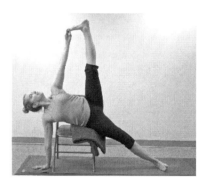

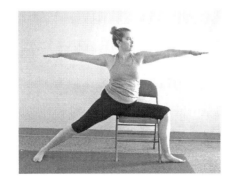 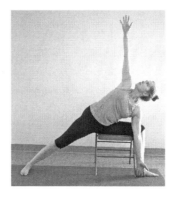 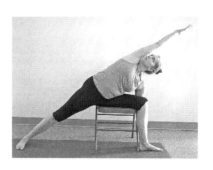

# NOTES

# SANSKRIT INDEX

# ENGLISH INDEX

## DELIA'S BIOGRAPHY

**Delia Quigley** is the Director of StillPoint Schoolhouse LLC. where she has been exploring and teaching how to live a holistic lifestyle, based on her 32 years of study, experience and practice. She is a certified Yoga instructor, holistic health counselor, whole foods Chef, photographer and author of eight books on yoga, meditation, nutrition, and cooking. She has hosted both radio and television programs, writes a food blog and is dedicated to maintaining her own daily practice.

Delia is the co-founder of the Ha-Tha Yoga Method, and the Chair Vinyasa Certification Program with Denise Kay. The Ha-Tha Yoga Method is an education based yoga training program offering professional instruction to further the growth of yoga practitioners. Our mission is to provide the highest level of instruction for yoga teachers, teachers-in-training, experienced yoga students, physical therapists, mental health counselors and health practitioners in the healing arts.

**Books by Delia:**

*Chair Vinyasa, Yoga Flow for Every Body*
*Empowering Your Life With Meditation*
*The Body Rejuvenation Cleanse*
*The Complete Idiots Guide to Detoxing Your Body*
*Super Charge with SuperFoods*
*Starting Over, Learning To Cook With Natural Foods*
*Cooking Healthy With One Foot Out The Door*
*Simply Smoothies*

**For more information:**
www.deliaquigley.com
www.ha-thayogamethod.com

73642799R00072

Made in the USA
Lexington, KY
10 December 2017